D0573477

get your body back
after baby

WEIGHT LOSS | NUTRITION | EXERCISE | RELATIONSHIPS | SEX | BREASTFEEDING

TRIUMPH
B O O K S

FROM THE EDITORS OF
FitPregnancy

Acknowledgments

SPECIAL PROJECTS EDITOR	JENNIFER CAROFANO
CREATIVE DIRECTOR	DONNA GIOVANNITTI
COPY EDITOR/RESEARCHER	MARIA S. VEGA
ASSISTANT ART DIRECTOR	TARA THOMPSON
PHOTO RESEARCHER	STACEY HARPER
DIRECTOR OF RIGHTS AND PERMISSIONS	FIONA MAYNARD

CONTRIBUTING WRITERS

Kim Schworm Acosta, Vanessa Geneva Ahern, Dagny Scott Barrios, Jennifer Barrett, Michele Bender, Sasha Brown-Worsham, Kate Neale Cooper, Julie Weingarden Dubin, Mona Gable, Kim Galeaz, Monica Gullon, Teri Hanson, Sara Jaye, Kathleen Kelleher, Alice Lesch Kelly, Carole Anderson Lucia, Marianne McGinnis, Colleen Moriarty, Christopher Napolitano, Pete Nelson, Kate Nolan, Lori Oliwenstein, Lorie Parch, Amy Paturel, M.S., M.P.H., Leigh Brown Perkins, Stephen Randall, Suz Redfearn, Tamekia Reece, Victoria Abbott Riccardi, Shari Roan, Elizabeth Rusch, Sarah Bowen Shea, Carrie Myers Smith, Mary Ellen Strote, Dana Sullivan, Laurie Tarkan, Robin Vitetta-Miller, M.S., Stacy Whitman

CONTRIBUTING PHOTOGRAPHERS

Reed Davis, Pascal Demeester, Getty Images, Lisa Hubbard, Jupiter Images, Catherine Ledner, David Martinez, Anthony-Masterson, Pornchai Mittongtare, Kana Okada, Victoria Pearson, Lisa Romerein, David Roth, Ted & Debbie, Elio Tolot, Romulo Yanes

This book is available in quantity at special discounts for your group or organization. For further information, contact:

TRIUMPH BOOKS
542 South Dearborn Street
Suite 750
Chicago, Illinois 60605
(312) 939-3330
Fax (312) 663-3557
www.triumphbooks.com

ISBN: 978-1-60078-364-7

Printed in USA

Contents

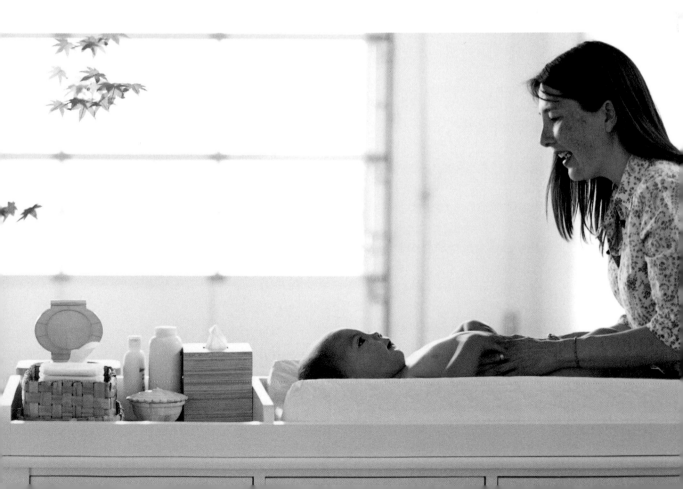

Congratulations! You've just had a baby.

Now, you want your body back. Easier said than done. At two weeks post-pregnancy you might wonder why you still look five months pregnant, but be patient: By six weeks your uterus should be back to its original size and most of the extra fluids you accumulated while expecting will be gone. The next steps? Losing the baby weight, regaining your prepregnancy shape and starting to feel like yourself again.

That's where *Fit Pregnancy's Get Your Body Back After Baby* can help. From making it through the first six weeks as a new mom—on less sleep and with little time to exercise—to eventually beginning (and maintaining!) a regular workout routine, in the pages to follow you'll find our best advice for shedding those extra pounds and strengthening the muscles most taxed during pregnancy.

You'll also uncover tips on eating healthy, including delicious—and easy to prepare—recipes with the nutrients you need. And, how about that sex life? Discover how to balance your relationship, both physically and emotionally, with your role as new mom.

Finally, you'll learn the basics of breastfeeding (a great way to burn calories!) as well as how to bond with your baby and, ultimately, become a confident mom. But remember: It took nine months to grow your baby and it will likely take that long to lose the baby weight. No worries: *Fit Pregnancy's Get Your Body Back After Baby* has plenty of tips, recipes and workouts that will help you get your body back— and, possibly, in even better shape than before.

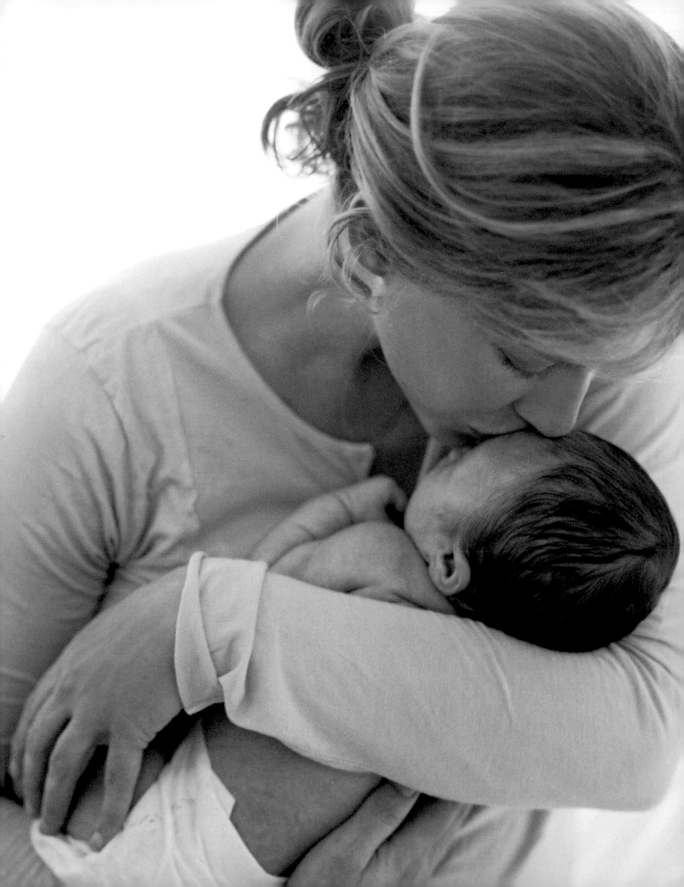

TAKING CARE OF YOU | 1

You've made it through pregnancy, labor and

delivery. You've got a beautiful new baby. What you didn't expect was how sore and tired you'd be after giving birth. What's more, taking care of a newborn is taking its toll on you, both physically and emotionally. As any mother will attest, those first six weeks can be overwhelming, exhausting and, in a word, hard.

To make it through, the most important thing you can do is take care of yourself. The following week-by-week guide to recovering after childbirth will help you gauge what's normal—and what warrants a call to your doctor. Plus, easy exercises designed to allay stress and strengthen the muscles most taxed during pregnancy and delivery will help you begin to feel like yourself again.

The key to recovering from childbirth and taking care of your newborn is to place nonessential activities on hold and take care of yourself, too. "Mothers think that because they're going home from the hospital, they're good to go," says Nancy Chandley-Adams, R.N., IBCLC, who works in the patient-education department at Women and Infants Hospital in Providence, R.I. "But their bodies still have to recover."

The key to recovery during your first six weeks postpartum is narrowing your to-do list down to the essentials. Easier said than done? Get down to basics with this week-by-week guide to taking care of yourself after you have a baby.

Week one

Giving birth impacts almost every part of your body. "Many new moms are surprised at how sore and tired they are," says Karen Ruby Brown, a certified nurse-midwife at the University of California, San Diego, Community Women's Health Program. Another surprise is how utterly "goopy" you feel. "The body is releasing so much stuff—blood, sweat, tears, milk—that women feel like walking bodily fluid factories," Brown explains. During week one you'll experience uterine contractions, bloody vaginal discharge, possible breast engorgement and post-episiotomy pain (if you had one). You'll pass clots that can be as large as a small plum. You'll feel even more uncomfortable and in pain if you had a Cesarean section. (For symptoms that require immediate medical attention, see "Red Flags," pg. 18.)

HOW TO CARE FOR YOURSELF

MAKE TIME TO MINIMIZE PAIN Strategies may include taking sitz baths, using hemorrhoid wipes, squirting the vaginal area with warm water (especially after going to the bathroom) and following your doctor's recommendations regarding incision sites. (For more information on recovering from a vaginal delivery or Cesarean section, see "Baby Your Body," pgs. 11 and 13.)

NURSE FREQUENTLY TO PREVENT BREAST ENGORGEMENT When your milk comes in, usually between days three and five, your breasts may become overfull, swollen and hard. You can relieve engorgement pain by applying ice packs or cold cabbage leaves. (The latter haven't been proved effective, but may work for some women.)

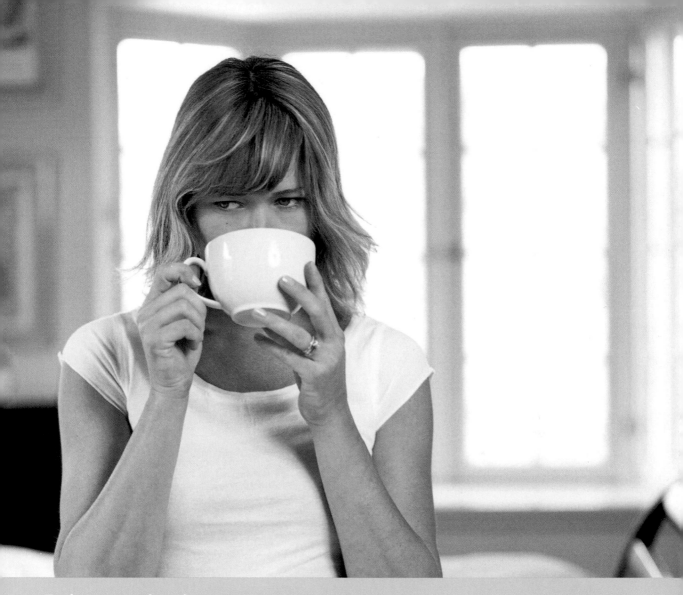

Baby your body
To ease your recovery from labor and delivery, rest as much as you can, drink plenty of fluids and keep taking your prenatal vitamin. Also follow these self-care tips:

If you had a vaginal delivery

KEEP IT CLEAN Be sure to shower daily if you had a perineal tear or episiotomy.

KEEP IT COMFY If you didn't have a perineal tear or episiotomy, it's safe to take a daily sitz bath (sit in 2 inches of warm water) to soothe your perineum and/or hemorrhoids. Also apply witch hazel pads to your nether region.

AVOID BATHS Wait to bathe until six weeks after delivery, when your cervix is fully closed.

KEEP IT MOVING To prevent constipation, request stool softeners before you leave the hospital. Try milk of magnesia if you haven't had a bowel movement in four days.

SAY YES TO DRUGS Ease post-delivery aches and pains with a heating pad and 800 milligrams (mg) of ibuprofen (Advil or Motrin) up to three times a day.

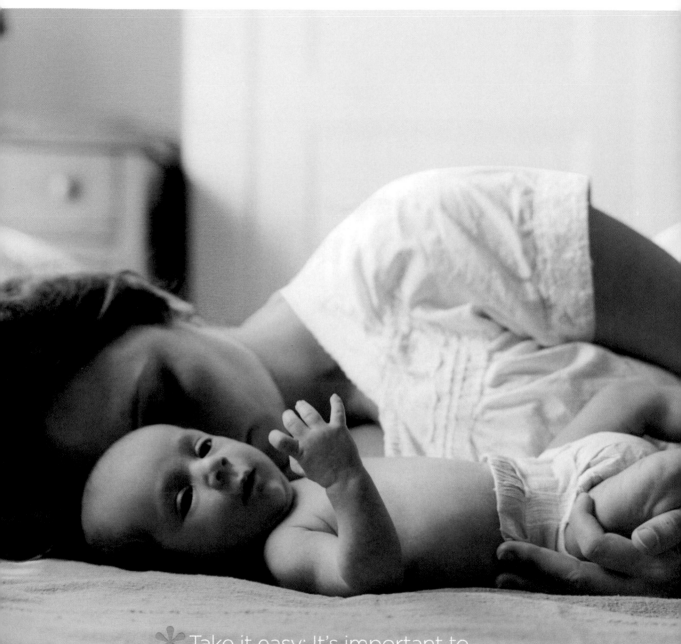

Take it easy: It's important to give your body time to recover after a Cesarean section.

If you had a Cesarean section

PLAN TO GET UP AND ABOUT "We suggest that patients get out of bed and start moving within 24 hours of a C-section because movement decreases the risk of blood clots and gets your digestive system functioning again," says Alison Edelman, M.D., M.P.H., an assistant professor of obstetrics and gynecology at Oregon Health & Sciences University in Portland. You'll need to start slowly and with help from your nurse, as you may be a bit dizzy when you first get up. Soon enough you'll be able to take a stroll around your hospital floor. The need to get back on your feet is one reason you should take the pain medicine your doctor prescribes.

You also can shower within a day of your surgery; doing so helps reduce the risk of infection. "Don't scrub your incision, but let the soapy water run over it," Edelman says. (Your bandages will likely be removed about 24 hours after surgery and replaced with small sticky bandages called Steri-Strips; it's fine if these get wet.) Dry the area by gently patting it or using a blow-dryer set on cool. It's safe to take a sitz bath when the incision has healed, generally seven to 10 days after surgery.

EXPECT UNEXPECTED PAIN Most women realize that they'll have pain after a C-section—it's major surgery, after all! But many are surprised by the intestinal spasms—OK, gas—they experience; this is a result of air becoming trapped in the abdomen during surgery. Getting out of bed and walking will help relieve gas pains. Additionally, your physician might also recommend taking simethicone tablets (Gas-X), which help alleviate gas and bloating. Also move your legs around while in bed—any bit of activity helps.

PREPARE TO TAKE IT EASY AT HOME "Don't drive for at least one week after a C-section delivery, limit stair climbing, and avoid heavy housework," says Henry Lerner, M.D., an OB-GYN in Newton, Mass., and a clinical instructor at Harvard Medical School. The age-old advice—don't lift anything heavier than your baby for two weeks—still stands. The staples that are commonly used to close the incision will probably be removed within three to seven days of delivery, but even then, it's important to avoid any strenuous activity for the first two weeks. Also pay attention to the following symptoms of infection; if you have any of them, call your doctor immediately: fever above 100.4° F; heavy vaginal bleeding; pain at the incision site that gets worse instead of better; blood or other fluid draining from your incision; or, reddened edges around your incision

EMBRACE YOUR BABY'S BIRTH For women who planned and hoped for a vaginal delivery, having a C-section can be emotionally devastating. If you just can't come to terms with your C-section, visit Postpartum Support International at postpartum.net. They'll guide you to support groups and even counselors who specialize in this area.

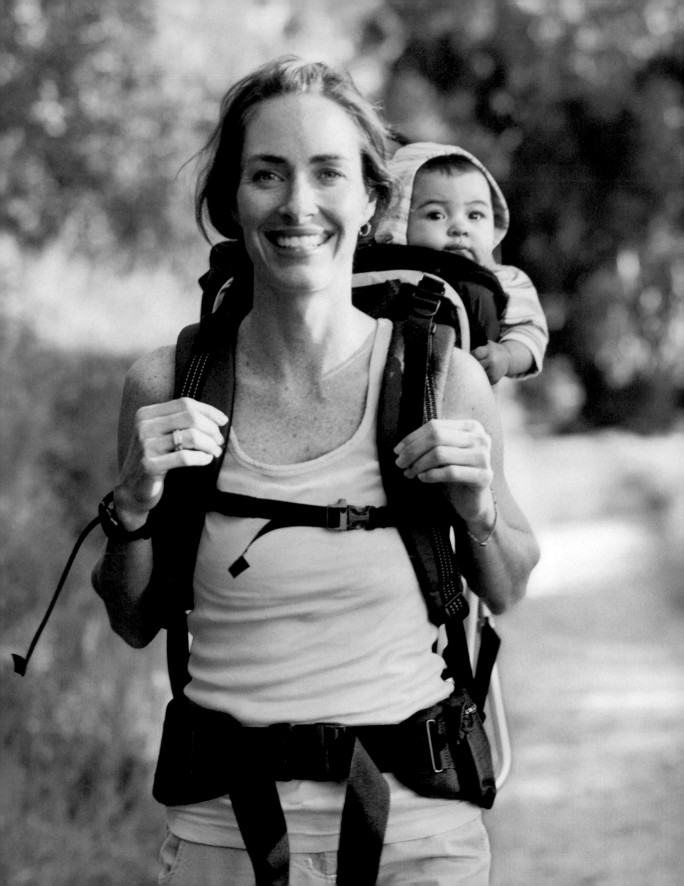

Week two

You'll start feeling better during week two, but that doesn't mean you should launch into major housecleaning mode. Instead, try to get outside. You'll continue to have vaginal discharge as well as soreness and itching at any incision sites. If you're breastfeeding, your nipples may be sore.

HOW TO CARE FOR YOURSELF

DON'T OVERDO IT Vaginal discharge, which was bright red during week one, will turn brown during week two. If you exert yourself too much, it will turn red again—that's a warning sign you're doing too much and need to slow down.

START TAKING BRIEF WALKS This will exercise your muscles and reduce your risk of developing blood clots, which are more common after childbirth. Take it easy, but do a little each day and increase the distance gradually.

GET HELP IF BREASTFEEDING HURTS Some nipple soreness is normal, but if they are cracked, bleeding or truly painful, contact a certified lactation consultant (Visit iblce.org, the International Board of Lactation Consultant Examiners).

✳ Taking walks will exercise your muscles and reduce your risk of developing blood clots.

Week three

During pregnancy, estrogen and progesterone levels are about 10 times higher than normal; once you give birth, they begin to plummet. By postpartum day seven they return to prepregnancy levels, but the emotional ups and downs are just starting. "Your hormones impact every organ system, and your body needs weeks to adjust," says OB-GYN Tracy W. Gaudet, M.D., director of integrative medicine at the Duke University School of Medicine in Durham, N.C. During this time your emotions can be all over the place.

HOW TO CARE FOR YOURSELF

DON'T SUFFER IN SILENCE Talk to your doctor, nurse or midwife as well as family and friends if you can't shake your moodiness, especially if you have a history of depression. (For more information, see "Avoid the Baby Blues," pg. 17.)

LOWER YOUR STANDARDS Give yourself a break if you don't measure up to prepregnancy expectations regarding housework and social obligations. When you're caring for a newborn, it's OK for the laundry to wait.

TAKE A BREAK EVERY DAY Do something special for yourself, even if you just call a friend, listen to music or read.

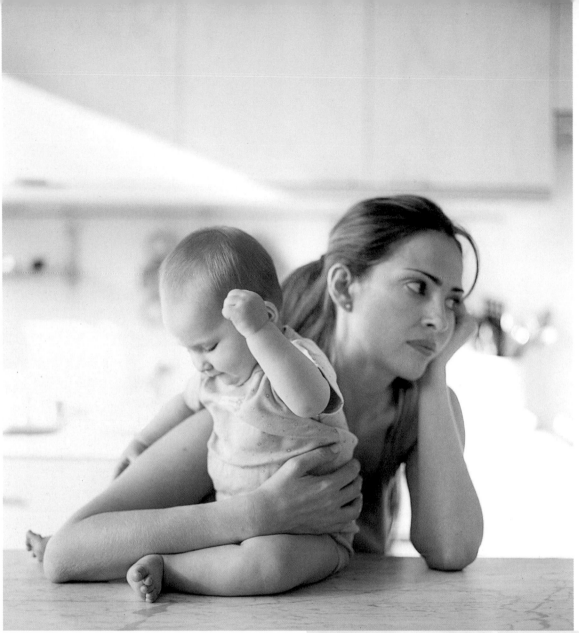

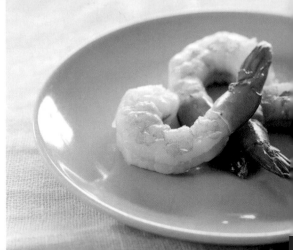

＊A daily dose of omega-3s can lower your risk for postpartum depression.

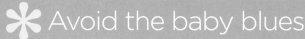 Avoid the baby blues

As many as 70 to 80 percent of new mothers experience the "baby blues," a mild change of mood beginning in the first few days after giving birth. Up to 10 percent develop true postpartum depression (PPD), according to the American College of Obstetricians and Gynecologists; women with a history of severe PMS, thyroid illness, or a personal or family history of depression are at increased risk. Symptoms of PPD include insomnia, loss of appetite, feeling emotionally disconnected from or resentful of your infant, memory loss and severe anxiety. "Postpartum depression is a very treatable illness, but getting to it quickly is important," says Diana Lynn Barnes, Psy.D., of Woodland Hills, Calif. Here are simple ways to help avoid PPD:

EAT OMEGA-3s One study found that countries in which people eat more omega-3-rich seafood had a lower rate of PPD. According to study author Joseph Hibbeln, M.D., a National Institutes of Health researcher, you should get 1 gram of omega-3s a day; sardines, cooked salmon, shrimp, avocados and flaxseed oil are all good sources (3 ounces of sardines provide about 1.3 grams). Fish-oil capsules—which contain only trace amounts of mercury—also are a good way to supplement your diet, according to Hibbeln.

SNOOZE It's tempting to catch up on daily tasks while the baby is sleeping, but don't. "One of the major risk factors for postpartum depression in new moms is sleep deprivation," says PPD expert Barnes.

GET ACTIVE "Exercise is a natural mood booster that can improve psychological health by relieving stress," says Kelli Calabrese, M.S., a lifestyle and weight management consultant in Flower Mound, Texas. The company of others during exercise also helps. "Postpartum exercise classes or mommy-and-me groups that allow women to reach out to other women can be reassuring and lessen the possibility of depression," Barnes says.

PLAN BABY-FREE TIME "Make sure you get some time alone as a new mom, whether it's to practice yoga, meditate, write in a journal or even just take a bath at the end of the day," Barnes advises. "And don't feel guilty about it."

GET HELP While most mothers experience the "baby blues," if these feelings intensify or persist beyond a few weeks, call your doctor right away. You may be suffering from PPD. Or contact these organizations: Postpartum Support International (800-944-4PPD, postpartum.net) or Postpartum Education for Parents (805-564-3888, sbpep.org).

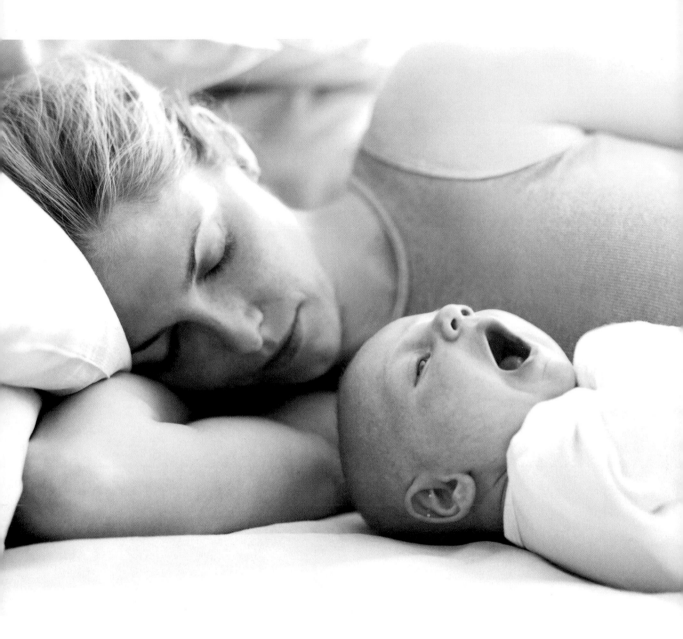

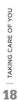 **Red flags** Contact your OB-GYN or midwife if you experience any of the following during your first six weeks postpartum:

- Hot or reddened breasts, with fever, chills or headache
- Foul-smelling discharge from the vagina or an incision site
- Loss of control over bowels or bladder
- Unexplained swelling, leg pain, chest pain, vomiting or fever

Week four

Your body has done a lot of healing by week four, but your brain may be foggy with exhaustion. "Never in your life will you be as sleep deprived as you are when you have a new baby," says Alice D. Domar, Ph.D., executive director of the Domar Center for Mind/Body Health in Boston. "But remind yourself that this phase of your life is temporary."

HOW TO CARE FOR YOURSELF

SLEEP WHENEVER YOU CAN Remind yourself to put everything but the most essential tasks on hold (e.g., leave the dirty dishes for later), nap when the baby does and sleep close to your baby so you can get maximum rest.

GET DAD'S HELP WITH FEEDING If you're nursing, once breastfeeding is established (after about a month or so), have your partner give the baby a bottle of pumped milk during the night so you can sleep.

PRACTICE STRESS-RELIEF TECHNIQUES Try meditation, a mindfulness exercise or a mini-relaxation: inhale slowly and deeply, hold for a couple of seconds, then exhale slowly and fully. (For three effective stress-relieving exercises, see "Stretch Away Stress," pg. 22.)

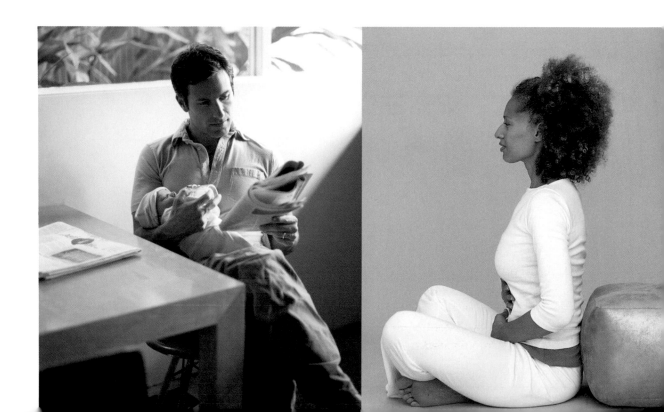

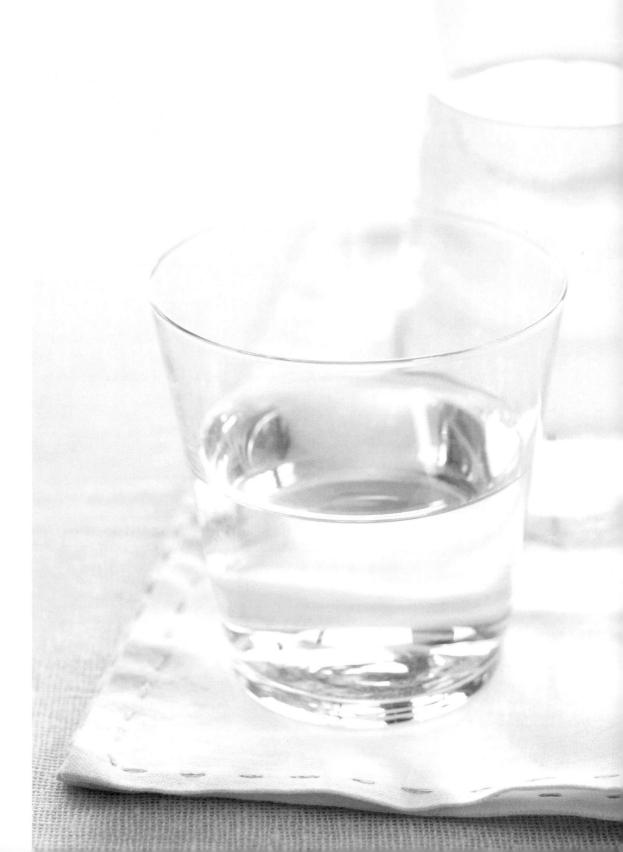

✳ Breast milk is 87 percent water. Be sure to drink eight or more glasses each day.

Week five

Although you are mostly healed, parts of you still feel strange. You may be leaking urine, itching from hemorrhoids or struggling with constipation. You wonder if your body will ever return to normal—you feel fat, your belly is poochy, your breasts are huge, and even the smallest amount of physical activity seems to wear you out.

HOW TO CARE FOR YOURSELF

START TAKING LONGER WALKS Daily exercise burns calories, tones muscles, improves mood and gets you out of the house. Don't want to leave your baby? Put her in a front carrier or stroller and take a walk together.

MAKE EVERY CALORIE COUNT Pack your diet with fresh fruits, vegetables, whole grains, nonfat dairy and low-fat protein. A peanut butter sandwich on whole-wheat bread with an apple and a glass of milk is a perfectly nutritious meal that takes only a few minutes to prepare.

DRINK PLENTY OF WATER It boosts your milk supply, helps your digestive system function effectively and fills you up.

BE PATIENT WITH YOUR BODY "Some women may feel completely recovered within a couple of weeks, but for others this process may take a good deal longer," Brown says.

Week six

Your body's (finally!) returning to normal. In fact, at your six-week checkup your doctor has probably given you the OK to start having sex again and return to work. But your life is completely different now that you've had a baby.

  "Becoming a mother often triggers women to re-evaluate who they are and their course in life," OB-GYN Gaudet says. "It's a hugely transforming event."

HOW TO CARE FOR YOURSELF

KEEP A JOURNAL Writing helps you examine and understand your emotions and find answers to difficult questions.

TALK WITH OTHER NEW MOTHERS Share thoughts and ideas with friends or women you meet in play groups, postpartum support groups or mom-baby exercise classes.

MAKE BIG DECISIONS CAREFULLY You're experiencing one of the most dramatic life transitions—it's not a good time to quit your job, leave your husband or move cross-country.

Stretch away stress

Three easy moves to strengthen and relax your overworked muscles.

Does your body ache? If so, it's not surprising. The daily responsibilities as a new mother can take a toll on your body, probably more than any other job you've ever had in your life. Constant lifting (of the car seat, stroller, baby, etc.), breastfeeding and diaper changing, coupled with heavier-than-normal breasts and weakened abdominal muscles, can all add up to a strain on your body's natural alignment. The result is that you feel tired and achy all day long.

The following moves are so gentle they can be done as early as the day after you deliver. Repeat them throughout the day as needed, holding each stretch for three full breaths. Remember to breathe in through your nose and out through your mouth. Always check with your doctor before starting any new exercise program.

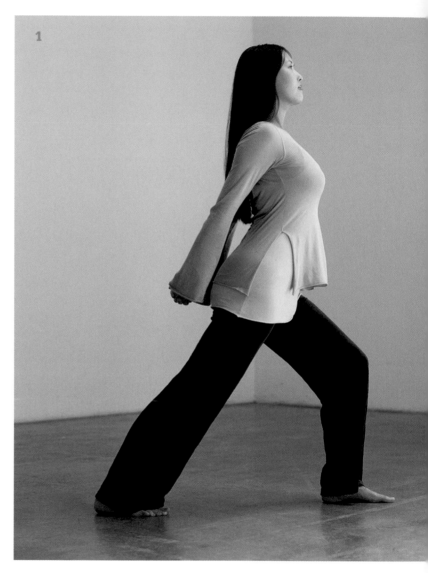

1

1 CHEST, CALF AND HIP STRETCH Stand with feet hip-width apart, then take a step back with your right foot, toes pointing straight ahead, right heel down. Lace your hands together behind your lower back, lifting your chest as you take a deep breath (Remember to breathe in through your nose and out through your mouth). Keeping shoulders relaxed, lengthen your torso as you bend your left leg, keeping your knee in line with your ankle, buttocks tight and abs drawn in [shown]. Switch sides and repeat.

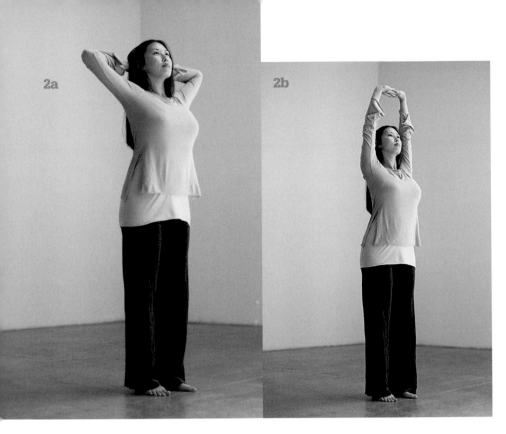

2a 2b

2
CHEST OPENER
Stand with feet hip-width apart and lace your hands behind your head, elbows wide. Breathe deeply in through your nose and out through your mouth. Gently press your head into your hands [A]. Straighten arms, palms up, and lean back slightly, keeping your thighs and buttocks firm [B].

✳ Try doing this routine every day and you may feel a lot more relaxed, invigorated and refreshed.

3 LOWER-BACK STRETCH
Stand with feet hip-width apart, knees bent, hands on thighs, fingers facing in. Lean forward from hips and point your tailbone back to straighten your spine [A]. Inhale, then exhale as you round your back like a cat, drawing your abs in and bringing chin toward chest [B].

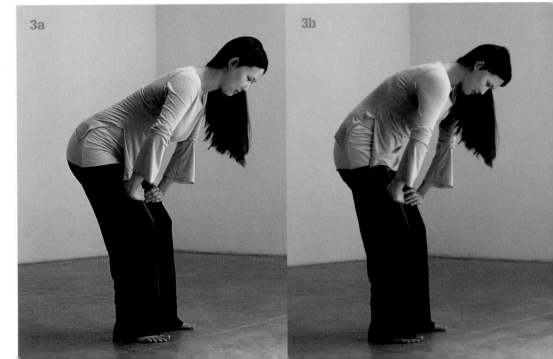

3a 3b

Brand-new mom moves

Help your body recover and get energized with moves so gentle you can do them the day after you deliver.

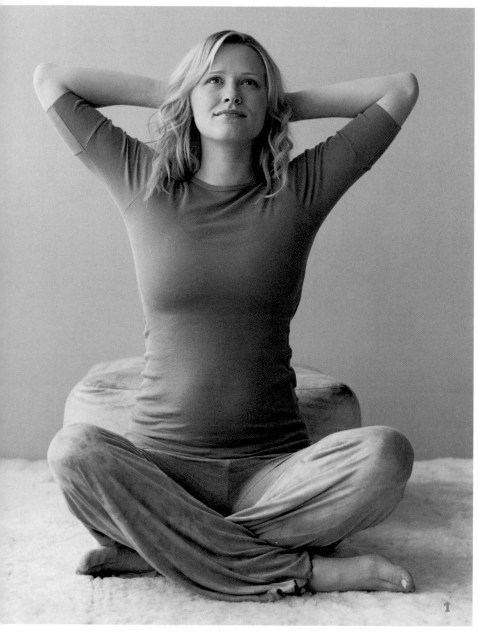

Pregnancy and childbirth put a strain on your body, leaving you feeling out of shape and low on energy. But, gentle moves that encourage deep breathing can help you feel like yourself again. The following workout, designed by Jennifer Gianni, an Asheville, N.C.-based specialist in prenatal and postpartum Pilates, incorporates deep breathing and increases circulation, which in turn will help to speed your recovery.

The moves are safe to do after a vaginal or Cesarean delivery and are so gentle that you can start them the day after you give birth (with your doctor's OK). Begin with the first move and slowly build your strength until you can complete the program. Start with five repetitions of each move, gradually working up to 10.

1 CHEST AND SHOULDER OPENER Sit comfortably with your legs crossed and lean back against a cushion or pillows. Lace your fingers behind your head, opening your elbows wide. Sit tall and lean back slightly, lifting your chest as you take a breath, slowly and deeply, until your ribcage expands [shown]. Exhale slowly and relax.

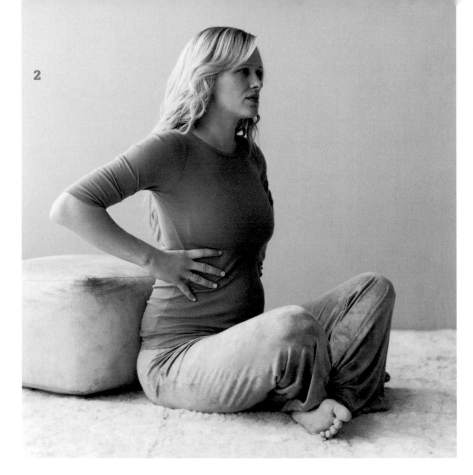

2 RIBCAGE BREATHING

Sit in a comfortable position, legs crossed, and lean back against a cushion or pillows. Lightly place your hands on your torso, just under your breasts, spreading your fingers wide along your ribcage. Inhale slowly and deeply through your nose, feeling your ribcage expand under your fingers. Exhale through your mouth as you gently draw your abs in [shown] and do a Kegel (See "Do Your Kegels," pg. 27).

✳ Gentle exercises will help you feel better.

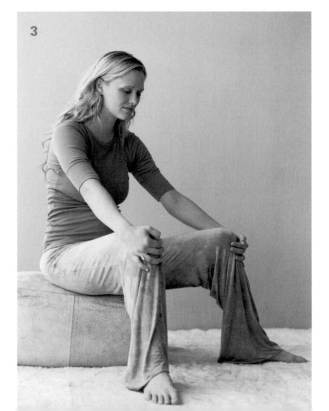

3 GENTLE PELVIC TILTS

Sitting erect on the edge of a chair, bed or cushion, place your hands on your knees. Inhale deeply through your nose as you lift your chest and lengthen your neck. Exhale slowly through your mouth as you round your spine, gently tucking your pelvis under and drawing your abs in [shown] as you do a Kegel. Return to starting position.

4

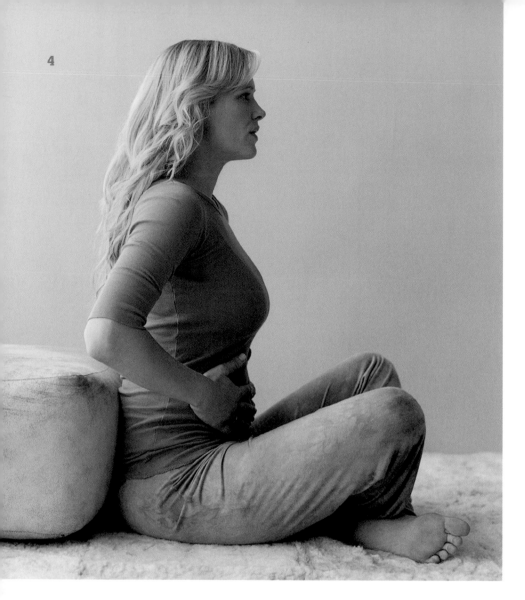

DRAWING IN Place your hands on your belly. Inhale slowly through your nose, expanding your belly, then exhale through your mouth and gently draw your abdominal muscles in, away from your hands, as you do a Kegel [shown]. Slowly release and repeat.

PELVIC TENSIONS

Lie on your back without arching it, knees bent and feet flat on the floor. Inhale through your nose, then exhale through your mouth, gently drawing in your abdominals. Slightly squeeze your glutes (buttocks) without lifting your hips [shown]. Slowly release and repeat.

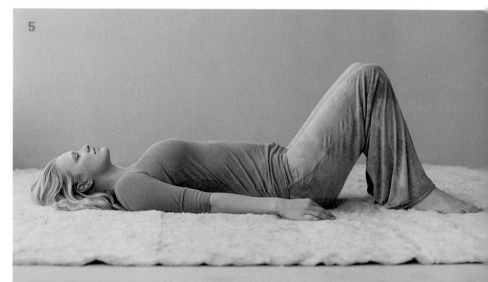

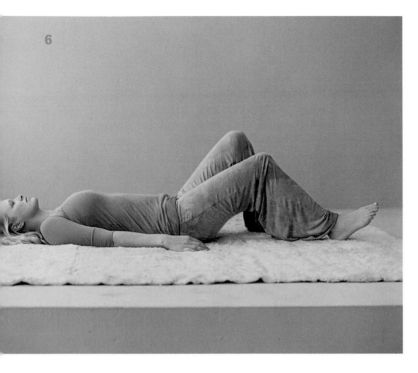

6

TOE WIGGLES AND LEG SLIDES Lying in pelvic tensions position, do 10 toe wiggles and ankle rolls with each foot to loosen your muscles. Next, keeping your heels on the floor, inhale through your nose and exhale through your mouth as you slide one heel away from you until your leg is almost straight [shown]. Slide the heel back and repeat with the other leg.

Do your Kegels

Kegels strengthen the pelvic-floor muscles around the vagina, promote healing after childbirth and help prevent urinary incontinence. To do a Kegel, inhale through your nose and, as you exhale through your mouth, contract the muscles surrounding the vagina as if you're holding back a stream of urine. Hold for 2 counts, breathing normally, then slowly release for 2 counts. Work up to holding the contraction for a count of 10. Repeat 10 times, 3 or 4 times a day. Kegels are most effective when done regularly.

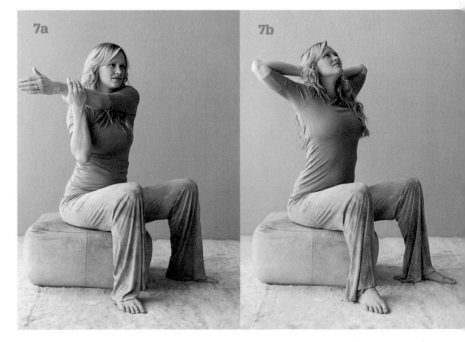

7 **UPPER-BODY STRETCHES** Cross your left arm over your chest and hold it with your right hand, keeping shoulders relaxed [A]. Hold for 2 breaths and switch sides. Then, clasp your hands behind your head, look up and keep your spine as long as possible, opening your chest [B]. Hold for 2 breaths and release.

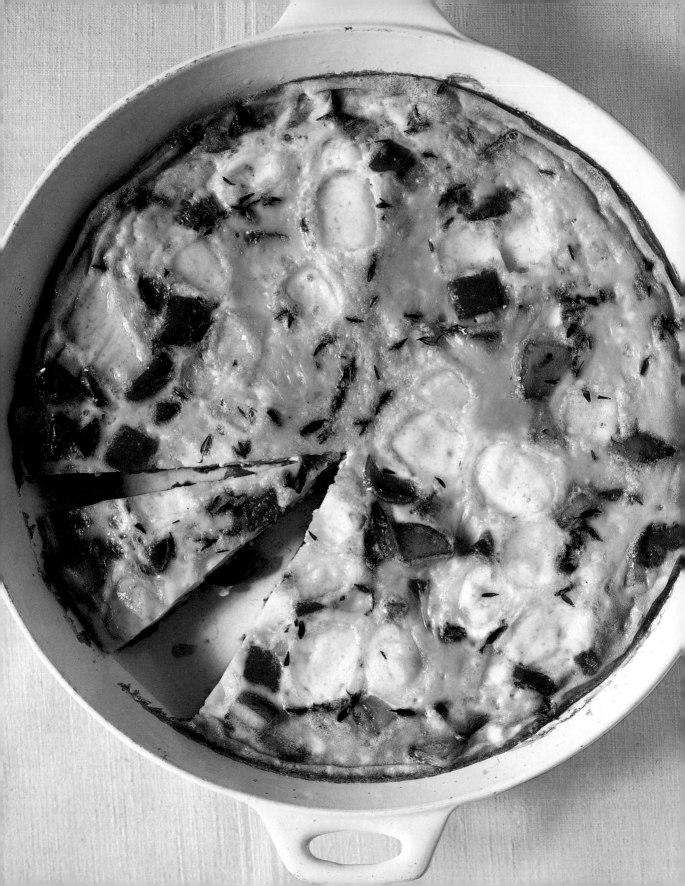

NUTRITION AND WEIGHT LOSS | 2

As a new mother, eating good-for-you food is

fundamental. Well-balanced nutrition is crucial to helping your body heal, keeping your energy level up and, if you're breastfeeding, passing essential nutrients along to your baby. Eating well, especially in the first few months after giving birth, also plays a critical role in helping to lose those post-pregnancy pounds.

From being aware of portion sizes to the importance of getting enough fluids and fiber, the following nine nutrition and weight-loss tips will help you make smart food choices and shed the baby weight. Plus, our one-day meal plan and easy-to-make recipes will ensure you're getting the nutrition you need in every delicious bite.

Healthful eating is important for everyone, but it's especially crucial if you've just had a baby. "The eating patterns you set in the first six months after having a baby can help you lay a foundation of healthful eating for the rest of your life," says Eileen Behan, R.D., a dietitian in New Hampshire and the author of the 2007 book *Eat Well, Lose Weight While Breastfeeding: The Complete Nutrition Book for Nursing Mothers*. We asked Behan and other experts for their top nutrition and weight-loss tips for new moms. Start following them now and you'll be well on your way to a healthier and trimmer you.

Know your needs

Simply navigating life with a newborn is tiring enough—who has the time (or energy) to put together a complicated meal plan? The good news is you don't have to; simply focus on getting adequate amounts of the nutrients below while paying attention to your calorie intake, and good health and a smaller waistline are within your reach.

"All these nutrients are vitally important if you've just had a baby," says Behan. "Calcium is vital for bone health; folate is important for future pregnancies and may protect you against heart disease; iron will help with anemia; protein is crucial for building and repairing your body's tissues; and vitamin C is necessary for iron absorption. You need even more of some of these nutrients during lactation to help with milk production—and because they leave your body with the milk." (Calorie needs vary depending on age, metabolism and exercise level.)

Here are guidelines to the calories and other nutrients you need daily for safe weight loss and good nutrition:

Nutrient guidelines

nutrient	breastfeeding	not breastfeeding
CALORIES	2,200-2,400	1,900-2,200
CALCIUM	1,000-1,300 mg	1,000-1,300 mg
FOLIC ACID	500 mcg	400 mcg
IRON	9-10 mg	8-18 mg
PROTEIN	71 g	46 g
VITAMIN C	115-120 mg	75 mg

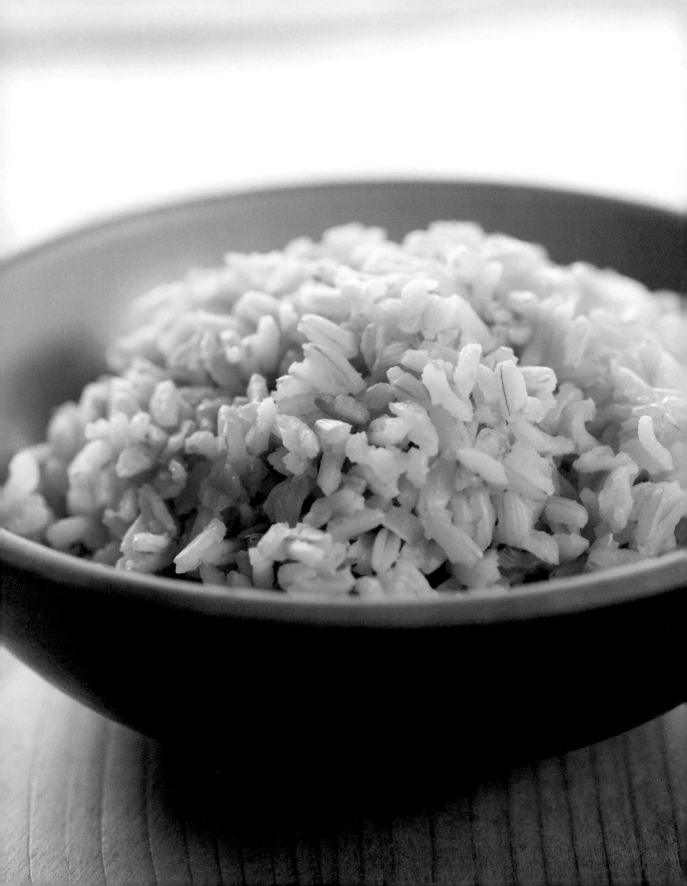

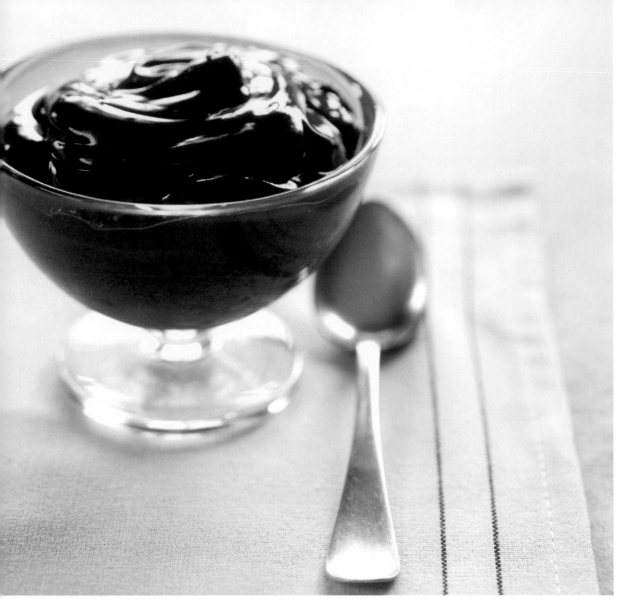

✳ Ready-to-go snacks

Cooked whole grains such as brown rice

Low-fat deli meats

Low-fat or fat-free pudding

Low-fat and fat-free yogurt

Prepackaged sliced fruits and vegetables

Ready-made salads

Whole-grain cereals, breads and pastas

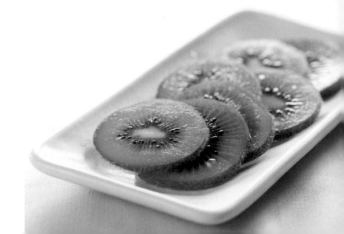

One-handed snacks

We know you've got your hands full these days, so reach for one of these healthful, baby-friendly treats when your belly starts to rumble.

- 1 toasted wedge of a whole-wheat baguette topped with 1 slice beefsteak tomato and 2 tablespoons crumbled feta cheese
[148 CALORIES, 5 G FAT]

- 1 whole-wheat English muffin with 1 tablespoon apple butter
[165 CALORIES, 1 G FAT]

- ½ cup low-fat cottage cheese with ¼ cup diced pineapple
[99 CALORIES, 1 G FAT]

- ½ whole-wheat pita with 2 tablespoons prepared hummus
[137 CALORIES, 4 G FAT]

- 1 cup grapes mixed with ½ cup low-fat vanilla yogurt
[166 CALORIES, 2 G FAT]

- 5 baby carrots dipped in ¼ cup black bean dip
[86 CALORIES, 0 G FAT]

- 2 part-skim mozzarella string cheese sticks
[100 CALORIES, 3 G FAT]

- 2 hard-boiled eggs with salt-free garlic and herb seasoning
[155 CALORIES, 11 G FAT]

- 2 tablespoons reduced-fat cream cheese spread in 1 large celery stalk
[79 CALORIES, 5 G FAT]

- ¼ cup low-fat granola
[105 CALORIES, 1 G FAT]

- 1 sliced zucchini dipped in ¼ cup reduced-fat blue cheese dressing
[109 CALORIES, 3 G FAT]

Stock up on healthful fast foods

When you're tired, short on time and hungry, it's tempting to reach for a bag of chips and a soda—if they're handy. So don't keep them around. "You want to be able to open the refrigerator door and grab something healthful that's ready to go," Behan says. (See "Ready-to-go Snacks," pg. 32.)

With healthy foods readily accessible, you'll snack less on chips, candy or white-flour-based, highly processed munchies, such as cookies and cakes. "They're usually high in salt and low in fiber," Behan says. "They're also irresistible, and it's easy to eat an enormous amount."

No time to grocery shop? Ask friends, neighbors and relatives to take turns bringing you healthful food from your list every few days. This way, you'll take care of your nutritional needs and get a dose of companionship—a godsend in those first few weeks. "Yes, nutrition is important," says Mavis Schorn, Ph.D., C.N.M, director of the nurse-midwifery educational program at the Vanderbilt University School of Nursing in Nashville, Tenn. "But so is having some social interaction, if only for 10 to 15 minutes."

Eat often, eat enough

Behan recommends that all new moms try to eat three healthy meals, plus two to three high-quality snacks per day (For inspiration, see our easy-to-follow one-day meal plan on pg. 35). Here's why eating frequently is important:

IF YOU'RE BREASTFEEDING, you need enough calories to fuel milk production. "It's very important for breastfeeding moms to get enough calories to make breast milk, the baby's sole source of nutrition," says Cheryl Lovelady, Ph.D., R.D., a professor of nutrition at the University of North Carolina at Greensboro. To ensure adequate milk production, you'll need to drink lots of water, too.

YOU NEED FUEL When you skip meals, your blood-sugar and energy levels drop. Eating often will help keep your energy up at a time when it's probably pretty low.

IT WILL HELP YOU LOSE WEIGHT "You have to eat well and often if you want to lose weight, or you'll be hungry all the time," Behan says. Being ravenous leads to bad choices.

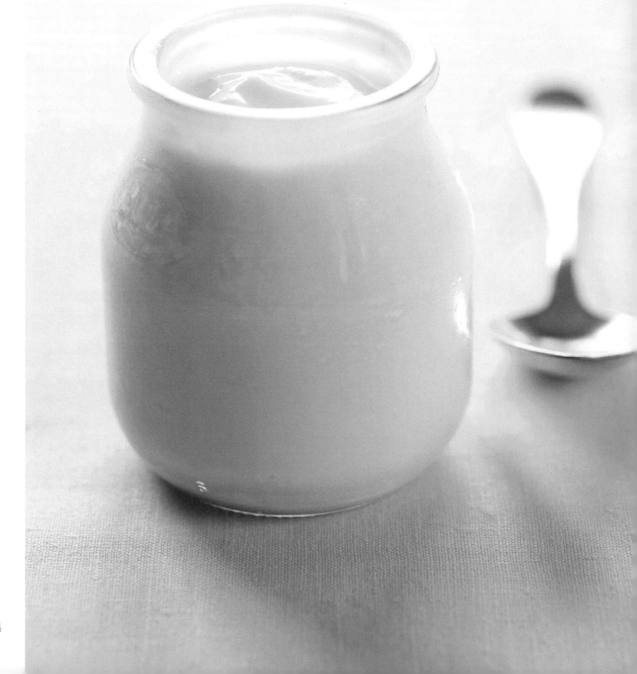

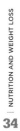

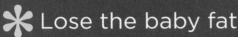

✱ Lose the baby fat

Get all the nutrients you need—and shed pounds—with this delicious one-day meal plan.

Breakfast
BROWN SUGAR-CINNAMON
OATMEAL WITH RAISINS
Combine in a microwave-safe bowl: ½ cup quick-cooking rolled oats; 1 cup low-fat (1%) milk; 2 tablespoons raisins; 1 teaspoon brown sugar; and ¼ teaspoon ground cinnamon. Microwave on high 1–2 minutes, or until liquid is absorbed; stir before serving.
1 medium banana
8 ounces orange juice

Midmorning snack
NUTS AND FRUIT
⅓ cup blanched almonds
¼ cup dried apricots

Lunch
ROAST BEEF WRAP WITH BASIL PESTO
Top one whole-wheat tortilla with 2 teaspoons prepared basil pesto, 3 ounces lean roast beef, 1 ounce reduced-fat Swiss cheese, 2 leaves romaine lettuce and 3 slices ripe tomato; roll up.
1 cup reduced-sodium tomato soup

Midafternoon snack
YOGURT AND FRUIT
8 ounces low-fat fruit yogurt
1 apple or pear

Dinner
SOY-GINGER GLAZED CHICKEN
WITH ROASTED SWEET POTATO
Combine in a small bowl: 1 tablespoon reduced-sodium soy sauce; 1 teaspoon honey; 1 teaspoon sesame oil; and ¼ teaspoon minced fresh ginger. Coat a shallow baking pan with cooking spray; place one 4-ounce skinless, boneless chicken breast in pan and coat with soy mixture.

Arrange one peeled, cubed sweet potato alongside; coat potato with cooking spray and season with salt and black pepper. Roast at 400˚F for 30–35 minutes or until chicken is cooked through and potato is fork-tender.

GARLIC-SPIKED SPINACH
Heat 2 teaspoons olive oil in a large skillet; add one minced garlic clove and cook 1 minute. Add 4 cups baby spinach leaves; cover and steam 30 seconds or until spinach wilts. Season to taste with salt and pepper.
1 whole-grain roll with 2 teaspoons light butter

Dessert
STRAWBERRY-KIWI SMOOTHIE
In a blender, combine 1 cup low-fat (1%) milk, ½ cup sliced strawberries and one peeled, sliced kiwi; purée until smooth.

[Nutrition score]
The calorie count for this meal plan is 2,272 calories, 27% fat (70 g; 17.4 g saturated, 26 g monounsaturated, 10.7 g polyunsaturated), 55% carbohydrate (331 g), 18% protein (108 g), 41 g fiber, 16.5 mg iron, 1,661 mg calcium, 396 mg vitamin C, 295 mcg folate, 1,945 mg sodium.

If you are not breastfeeding, stick to a diet that's closer to 1,900 calories. Modify this one-day meal plan by eliminating the almonds from the midmorning snack, 1 ounce of roast beef from the wrap and the buttered roll at dinner, and you'll be right where you should be nutrient-wise: 1,868 calories, 20% fat (41 g; 12.5 g saturated, 10.5 g monounsat-urated, 4.8 g polyunsaturated), 65% carbohy-drate (309 g), 15% protein (88 g), 34 g fiber, 14 mg iron, 1491 mg calcium, 396 mg vitamin C, 251 mcg folate, 1,671 mg sodium.

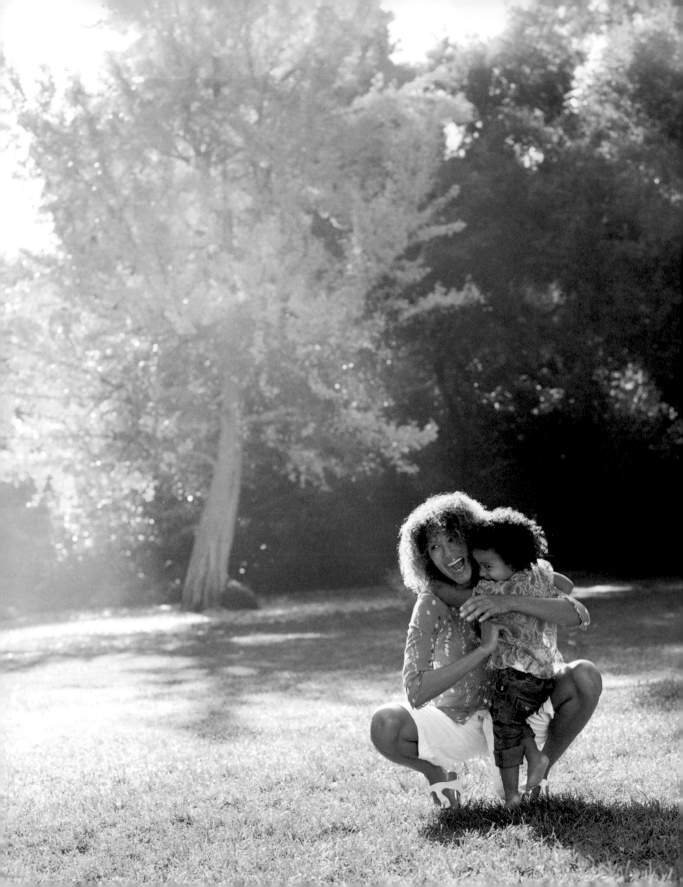

Pay attention to what your body says

Debra Waterhouse, R.D., M.P.H., a dietitian in Orinda, Calif. and the author of the 2003 book *Outsmarting the Female Fat Cell—After Pregnancy,* suggests that you ask yourself the following questions when you feel the urge to munch:

AM I HUNGRY? If so, give yourself permission to eat. If not, are you just tired or bored? Instead of eating, rest, call a friend, take a walk, play with your baby—just don't eat because you can't think of anything else to do.

WHAT AM I HUNGRY FOR? The more satisfied you are with what you eat, the less you'll eat and the better you'll feel. "If you crave chocolate ice cream but pick something healthier, you'll eventually break down and have the ice cream—after eating the yogurt, then the nuts, then the cheese," Waterhouse says. If you're craving something, go ahead and eat it—but opt for a small portion.

IS MY HUNGER SATISFIED? If it is—or almost is—stop eating. "Most people don't check in with themselves—they finish what's on their plate, and that's that, " Waterhouse says. "Instead, pause every five to 10 bites and see if you're eaten enough, if you're satisfied and if your stomach is full enough without being overly filled."

Be aware of portion sizes

Americans have become accustomed to supersized portions of everything from salad to soda. "Portion sizes have gotten out of control," nutritionist Lovelady says. Here's a quick rundown of serving sizes to aim for:

Food	Serving size
VEGETABLES	½ cup cooked or 1 cup raw
FRUIT	1 piece (or one cup); or ½-1 cup 100-percent juice
DAIRY (milk, yogurt, etc.)	8 ounces
PROTEIN	2–3 ounces
BREAD	1 slice
OLIVE OR CANOLA OIL	1 teaspoon
PASTA OR RICE	½ cup cooked

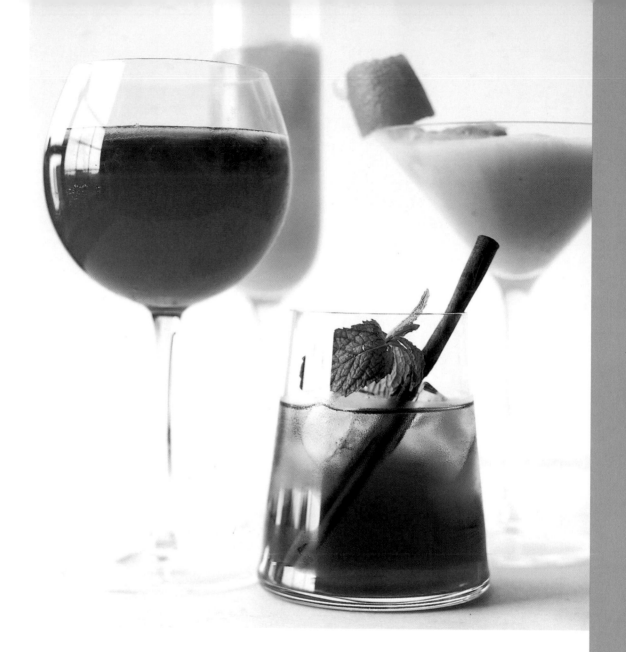

Load up on fluids and fiber

Constipation is a common problem for many women post-delivery. To prevent (or treat it), drink at least eight 8-ounce glasses of fluids a day—even more if you find yourself feeling thirsty, especially if you're nursing. Water is a good choice, but you also can opt for fat-free or low-fat milk, and up to 8 ounces a day of 100-percent fruit juices. In fact, virtually all liquids, including tea, soup and even the water in juicy fruit, count toward your quota, says Behan. (Smoothies are a fast, easy way to stay hydrated and get important vitamins and nutrients—all in a soothing drink. For delicious recipes, see "Super Smoothies," pg. 39.)

As for fiber sources: "The gold standard is fruit, veggies and whole grains, but sometimes that's not enough," says midwife Schorn. "If you're still having problems moving your bowels, try lemonade or warm liquids such as herbal teas. And if that fails, try grandma's old standby: prunes and prune juice."

Super smoothies

For each recipe, combine and blend ingredients until smooth. Each makes one 12-ounce serving.

CUCUMBER-CANTALOUPE COOLER

This refreshing drink delivers plenty of protein, calcium and vitamin C.

- ½ cup cucumber, peeled and cubed
- 1 cup cantaloupe, cubed
- ½ cup plain low-fat yogurt
- 4 fresh mint leaves, or to taste
- 8 ice cubes
- 1 tablespoon honey
- 1 teaspoon lemon zest

[Per serving] 223 calories, 18% fat (5 g), 69% carbohydrate (41 g), 13% protein (8 g), 4 g fiber, 14 mg iron, 291 mg calcium, 40 mcg folate, 73 mg vitamin C.

CARROT-CITRUS BOOSTER

Even if you don't like straight carrot juice, you'll enjoy this sweet drink.

- ¾ cup carrot juice
- ¾ cup lemon sorbet
- 8 ice cubes

[Per serving] 284 calories, 1% fat (less than 1 g), 97% carbohydrate (70 g), 2% protein (2 g), 2 g fiber, 1 mg iron, 44 mg calcium, 7 mcg folate, 26 mg vitamin C.

SOY FREEZE

Get all the benefits of soy in this sweet blend.

- ½ cup vanilla soy milk
- ½ cup low-fat vanilla frozen yogurt
- 1 medium banana, peeled
- ½ cup apricot juice
- 3 ice cubes

[Per serving] 396 calories, 16% fat (8 g), 76% carbohydrate (81 g), 8% protein (9 g), 7 g fiber, 2 mg iron, 126 mg calcium, 50 mcg folate, 22 mg vitamin C.

GINGER-PEACH PASSION

A touch of fresh ginger, as well as tropical mango, gives this peach blend a surprise twist.

- ½ cup peaches, peeled and sliced (or canned peaches, drained)
- 1 cup low-fat vanilla frozen yogurt
- ¼ cup mango juice
- ½ teaspoon grated fresh ginger

[Per serving] 320 calories, 22% fat (8 g), 70% carbohydrate (59 g), 8% protein (7 g), 2 g fiber, 1 mg iron, 217 mg calcium, 15 mcg folate, 11 mg vitamin C.

BANANA-BERRY DELIGHT

For the best texture, use only frozen berries when making this smoothie.

- 1 small banana, peeled
- 1 cup frozen mixed berries
- ½ cup vanilla soy milk
- 2 teaspoons lemon juice
- ½ cup low-fat vanilla frozen yogurt

[Per serving] 346 calories, 17% fat (7 g), 74% carbohydrate (69 g), 9% protein (8 g), 7 g fiber, 3 mg iron, 141 mg calcium, 61 mcg folate, 80 mg vitamin C.

TOMATO CRUSH

You'll get a blast of vitamin C from this light and tasty drink.

- ¼ cup vegetable juice, such as V8
- ½ cup orange juice
- 1 orange, peeled and sectioned
- 8 ice cubes

[Per serving] 134 calories, 2% fat (less than 1 g), 90% carbohydrate (32 g), 8% protein (3 g), 3 g fiber, 1 mg iron, 86 mg calcium, 85 mcg folate, 157 mg vitamin C.

Power punches

Healthy additions for any smoothie:

ALMONDS
2 tablespoons (ground) thicken smoothies while supplying protein, fiber, vitamin E and calcium.

SOY POWDER
2 tablespoons pack nearly half the protein you need every day.

TOFU
2 ounces of tofu that's processed with calcium sulfate add 200 milligrams of calcium, plus protein.

WHEAT GERM
2 tablespoons provide protein, fiber and folate.

Nursing nutrition in a glass

Staying hydrated is particularly important during breastfeeding to create an adequate milk supply, among other reasons. Lactating women also need more of vitamins A, C and E than during pregnancy; using different types of fruit as ingredients for your smoothie can provide at least some of these necessary vitamins. And, including milk, soy milk or yogurt can be one good way to help you reach your daily calcium quota of 1,000 milligrams.

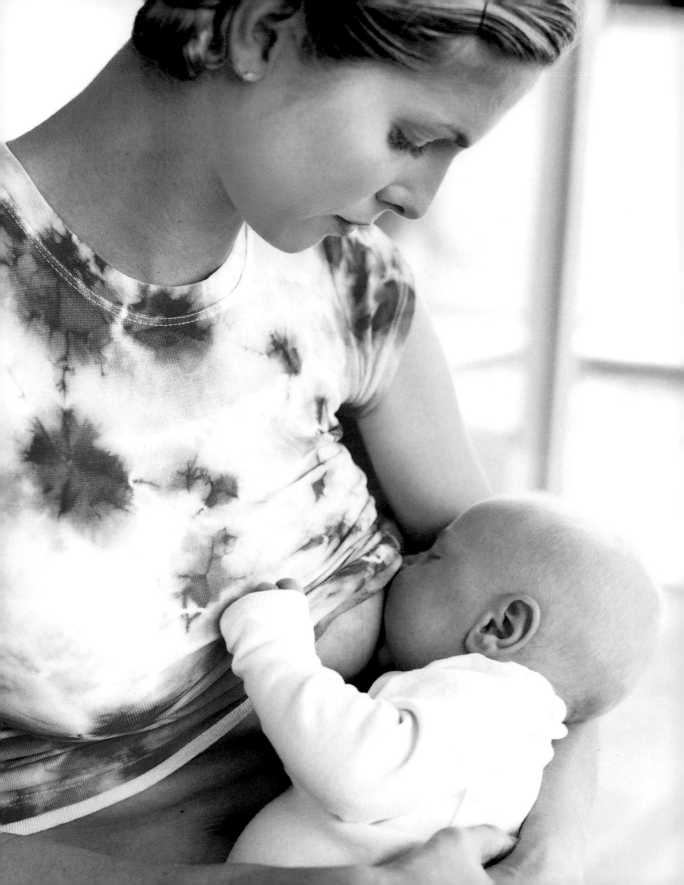

The secret to easy weight loss

How would you like to burn up to 500 calories a day and improve your baby's health, too? The secret is as old as childbirth itself: breastfeeding.

While nursing reduces the risk of many health risks for your baby, from ear infections to childhood cancers, there's also a correlation between nursing and reduced weight gain for you. In one study, women who had gained the least amount of weight eight years after having a baby were the ones who had breastfed exclusively for the longest period. (Exercise helps, too—these women also had begun and maintained an aerobic exercise program.)

A word of caution: Once your baby starts nursing less—usually at about 9 to 12 months, when solid foods are a regular part of the baby's diet—you'll need to decrease your calorie intake or you'll start putting on weight.

Avoid restrictive diets

The problem with most diets is simple but vexing: They cut calories so drastically that as soon as you've lost the weight and resume your normal eating patterns, the weight comes back—and then some. Some diets also restrict healthy carbohydrates (such as whole grains and fruit)—a no-no for many reasons. "Whatever you do, don't cut 'good' carbs," Waterhouse says. "Your body needs them in every way—they're typically fiber-rich, they help you feel full, and they're your brain's main energy source." But do cut simple carbs such as white pasta, bread and rice.

If you're hell-bent on following a specific plan, our experts say Weight Watchers is a reliable one because it emphasizes behavior modification and a slow weight loss of 1 to 2 pounds per week. They even have a plan for breastfeeding moms.

Take naps

"Getting plenty of sleep has been shown to help with weight loss because you're not compelled to binge on high-calorie, high-sugar foods for energy," says Sheah Rarback, M.S., R.D., director of nutrition at the Mailman Center for Child Development at the University of Miami's Miller School of Medicine. Strange sleep cycles like those forced on you by a newborn can upset your metabolism and make it harder for you to lose the pregnancy weight, Rarback says. Nap when the baby does if you need to, housework be damned. That way, you won't end up with a long-term sleep deficit, and you'll keep your energy levels—and cravings—in check.

Go easy on yourself

It can take a year or more to lose the pregnancy weight. "You need to think of pregnancy as an 18-month experience: nine months of gestation, nine months postpartum," Behan says. "This is a time when there's a lot happening—you're adjusting to your new life, your body is trying to replenish itself after pregnancy, you've gone through labor and delivery, and you may be breastfeeding. It's a lot to adjust to, so don't beat yourself up if you're not bouncing back as quickly as you'd like."

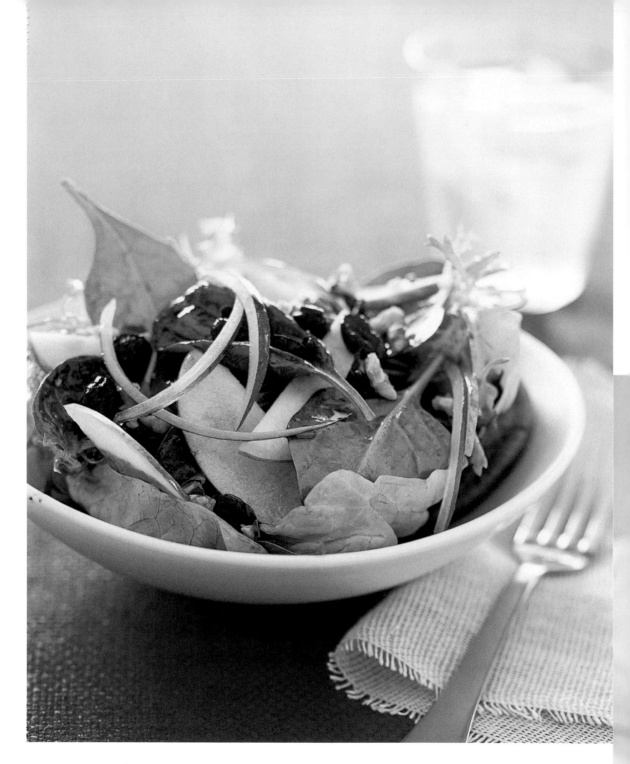

✳ Foods rich in fiber keep you feeling
full longer. Aim for 25 grams each day.

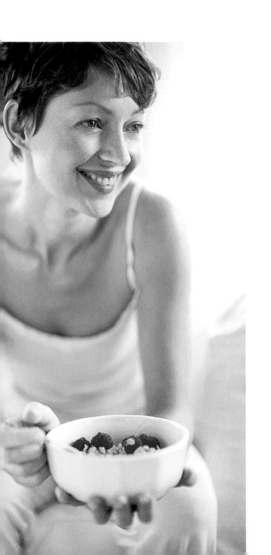

The benefits of fiber

As a new mom, it's more important than ever to get the 25 grams of fiber a day recommended for women by the American Dietetic Association. Fiber's contribution to post-baby weight loss is yet another benefit—and one that continues long after delivery.

The indigestible part of the carbohydrate in plants, fiber is found in fruits, vegetables, grains and legumes (beans and peas), though not in animal products such as dairy, meat or seafood. It's surprisingly easy to work fiber into your daily fare. "You don't have to seek out fancy foods or exotic ingredients to eat a high-fiber diet," says registered dietitian Tanya Zuckerbrot of New York City. "Almost everyone has a can of beans in the pantry."

Fiber comes in two forms: soluble and insoluble. Think of the former as a sponge and the latter as a broom. Soluble fiber, found in oats and beans, makes you feel full by absorbing water. It mixes food into a gel, soaking up cholesterol, fats and sugars before they enter the bloodstream (hence the "sponge" action). Insoluble fiber, which your grandmother called roughage, sweeps food through your digestive system (the "broom" effect); broccoli and whole-grain cereals fall into this category. Both types of fiber improve digestion and overall health.

Zippy plumbing is good, vigorous health is brilliant, but a slender waistline—especially after having a baby—really gets new moms' attention. Fiber helps here, too: It keeps you full but has no calories. Fiber also stabilizes blood-sugar levels, so you can avoid the energy spikes and crashes that commonly occur after eating empty, refined carbs such as white rice, processed snack foods and soda.

"Foods rich in fiber and water are great ways to fill up without filling out," says nutritionist Elizabeth Somer, M.A., R.D., of Salem, Ore. And what about the carbohydrate count in fiber? "A lot of people are afraid to add fiber to their diet because it's found in carbohydrate foods and they've been programmed to believe that carbs make you fat," Zuckerbrot states. "But it's the quality and quantity of carbs that matter. And the fact remains that fiber is also a powerful tool for weight loss."

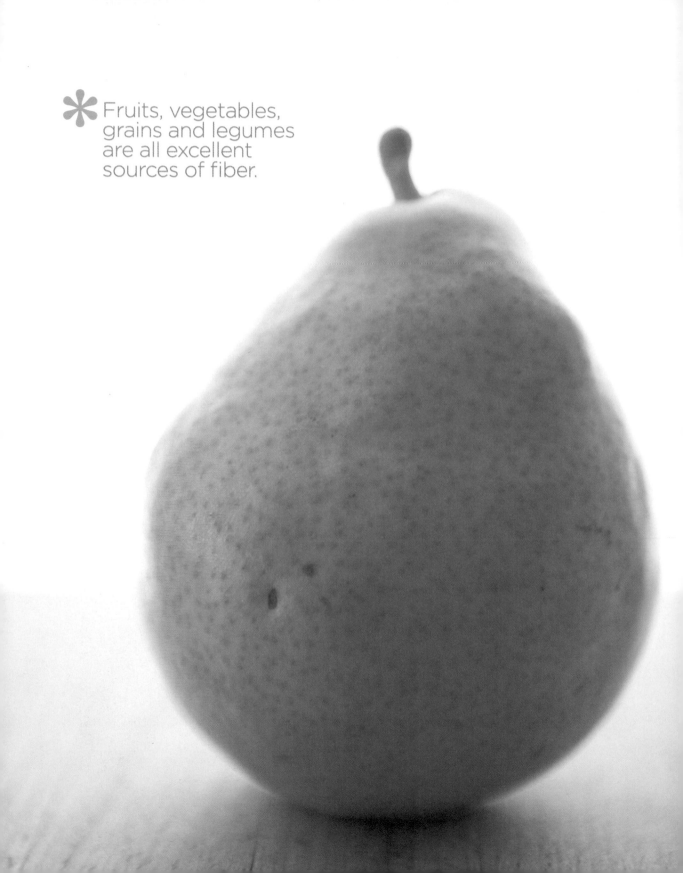

* Fruits, vegetables,
grains and legumes
are all excellent
sources of fiber.

Fiber fix

Boosting your fiber intake does not have to mean adding garbanzo beans to every meal. Just make creative adjustments to the menu you already love. Perk up salads with spinach and chopped vegetables, give smoothies a punch by adding extra berries or eat the skins of fruits and vegetables. If you're nursing, add fiber to your diet slowly, say an extra 2 to 5 grams a day; certain high-fiber foods may cause some babies to become gassy or fussy. (It may take experimentation to discover which foods cause discomfort or sit well with your baby.) Here are more great options for pumping up your roughage:

FOOD	FIBER (g)
Lentils (1 cup)	16
Split peas (1 cup)	16
Black beans (1 cup)	15
Collard greens (1 cup cooked)	15
Raspberries (1 cup)	8
Instant oatmeal (1 packet)	6
Pear (1 whole)	5
1 cup whole-wheat spaghetti	6
½ avocado	5
1 cup cooked broccoli	5
1 medium apple	4

In the rough

Although not technically a nutrient, fiber is an important part of a healthy diet—and even more so after having a baby. For most new moms, postpartum constipation is a normal occurrence as a result of dehydration (breastfeeding can deplete your body of liquids if you don't drink enough), inactivity and a departure from your regular diet (which often translates into a lack of fiber) in the weeks after childbirth. The solution? Getting enough fiber. The following fiber-rich recipes will help keep things moving smoothly.

SPICY ASIAN NOODLES

Serves 4
Prep time: 7 minutes
Cook time: 10 minutes

For dressing

1 tablespoon low-sodium soy sauce
2 tablespoons peanut butter
1 tablespoon tahini (sesame paste)
¼ cup hot water
1 tablespoon lime juice
1 tablespoon orange juice
1 teaspoon honey
Tabasco, to taste

For salad

8 ounces (½ pound) buck-wheat soba noodles
1 cup shredded carrots
1 cup red bell pepper strips
1 cup snow peas, rinsed
½ cup chopped scallions, green parts only
4 teaspoons chopped roasted peanuts
4 tablespoons chopped cilantro

Place dressing ingredients in a blender or food processor and blend until smooth. If mixture is too thick, thin with additional hot water, adding 1 tablespoon at a time. Set aside.

Prepare noodles according to package directions, rinse with cold water and drain. In a large bowl, toss noodles with dressing and carrots, red pepper, snow peas and scallions. Divide among four plates and garnish each with 1 teaspoon peanuts and 1 tablespoon chopped cilantro.

[Per serving] **(2 cups): 7 g fiber**

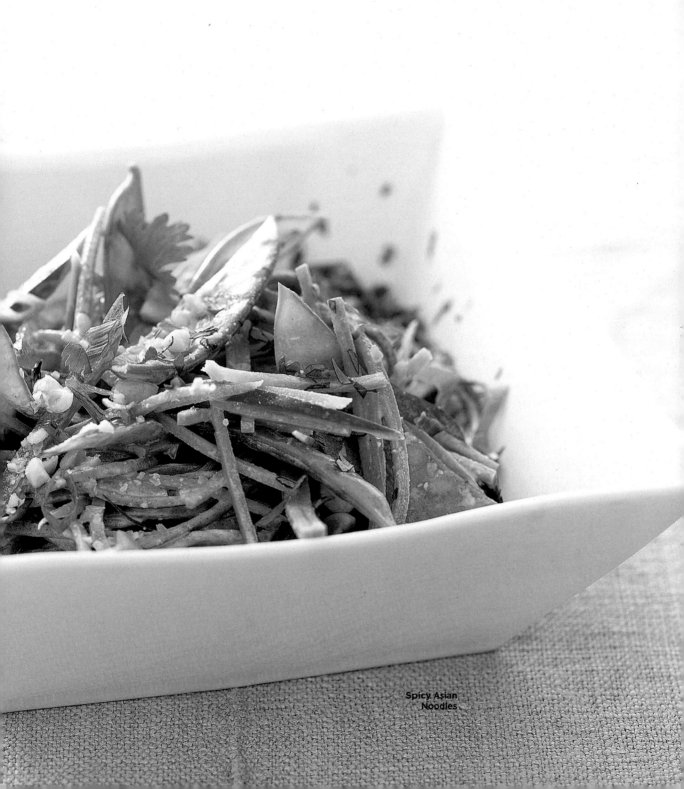

Spicy Asian
Noodles

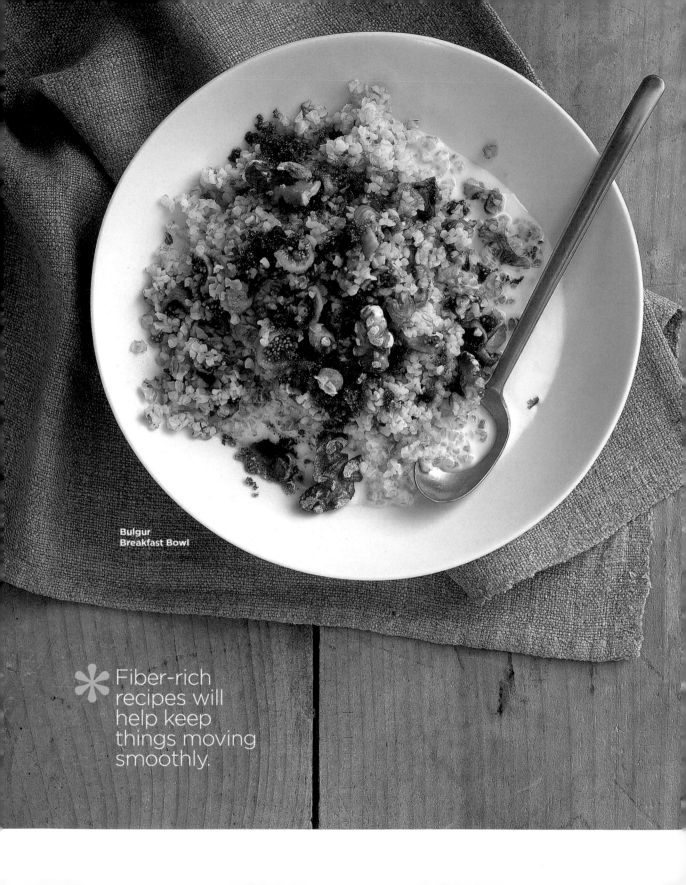

Bulgur
Breakfast Bowl

✳ Fiber-rich
recipes will
help keep
things moving
smoothly.

BULGUR BREAKFAST BOWL
Serves 6
Prep time: 5 minutes
Cook time: 15-18 minutes

$^3/_4$ cup coarse bulgur cereal
20 dried figs, coarsely chopped
$^1/_4$ cup chopped toasted walnuts
1 cup 2% milk
3 tablespoons brown sugar

Over high heat, bring a saucepan filled with water to boil. Add bulgur and cook until tender, about 15-18 minutes. Meanwhile, soften figs by soaking in a small bowl filled with very hot water.

Drain cooked bulgur and return to pot over low heat. Drain figs, squeezing out excess water, and stir into cereal. Add milk and sugar and stir, cooking briefly until sugar melts. Divide mixture among four bowls. Top each bowl with 1 tablespoon walnuts. Serve immediately.
[Per serving] (1 cup): **10 g fiber**

PASTA E FAGIOLE
Serves 4
Prep time: 5 minutes
Cook time: 15 minutes

Cooking spray
4 thin slices prosciutto
1 16-ounce can cannelloni (white) beans, rinsed and drained
1-2 cloves garlic, minced
$^1/_4$ cup julienned sundried tomatoes packed in oil
3 cups baby spinach
$^1/_2$ pound whole-wheat fusilli pasta, cooked according to package directions and drained (reserve $^1/_2$ of the cooking water)

Coat a large skillet with cooking spray and place over high heat. Cut prosciutto into pieces directly over the skillet. Fry prosciutto until edges are crispy, about 1-2 minutes. Add beans, garlic and sundried tomatoes; stir until ingredients are heated through, about 2 minutes. Add spinach; cook until just wilted. In a large bowl, toss pasta with bean mixture. To thin sauce, add the reserved cooking water slowly until desired consistency is reached. Serve immediately.
[Per serving] (1$^1/_2$ cups): **10 g fiber**

CHICKPEA SALAD
Serves 4
Prep time: 10 minutes
Cook time: 2-3 minutes

For dressing
2 tablespoons olive oil
2 tablespoons lemon juice
1 tablespoon water
$^1/_2$ teaspoon Dijon mustard
$^1/_2$ teaspoon dried mint
$^1/_2$ teaspoon dried oregano
1 garlic clove, minced
For salad
12 large leaves butter lettuce
  Cooking spray
2 large whole-wheat pitas, cut into small wedges
1 15-ounce can chickpeas, rinsed and drained
1 cup cherry tomatoes
20 kalamata olives
1 red bell pepper, chopped
1 cucumber, diced
$^1/_2$ red onion, chopped

In a small bowl, whisk together dressing ingredients and set aside. Next, line four shallow salad bowls with butter lettuce leaves.

Coat a large cast iron or non-stick skillet with cooking spray and place over high heat. Add pita wedges and toast, turning with tongs until golden, about 2-3 minutes. Reserve for tossing.

Place remaining ingredients in a large bowl and toss with dressing until well coated. Add toasted pita wedges and toss lightly. Divide equally among salad bowls. Serve immediately.
[Per serving] (2 cups): **9 g fiber**

New mom super foods

Eating the right foods post-pregnancy not only helps ensure that your baby gets crucial nutrients through your breast milk (if you're nursing), but a healthful diet also improves your own energy and emotional state, recovery from childbirth and short- and long-term health. "Some nutrient levels are depleted during pregnancy," says Megan Tubman, M.S., R.D., founder of Fresh Start Nutrition Studio in New York. "And if you're breastfeeding, you'll lose nutrients in your breast milk, too." The good news: Even if you're short on time (and what new mom isn't), replenishing lost nutrients is a snap when you eat plenty of these six power foods.

1. ALMONDS | **SERVING SIZE: 1 ½ OUNCES (OZ.)** All nuts are high in protein and fiber, but almonds also boast calcium, vitamin E, zinc and immune-boosting alpha-linolenic acid. "Vitamin E requirements are higher for breastfeeding moms, and it's a tough nutrient to get," says Melinda Johnson, M.S., R.D., national spokeswoman for the American Dietetic Association and owner of Nutrition for Slackers in Chandler, Ariz. Vitamin E, an antioxidant, helps protect against environmental damage to your body's cells.
TIPS Sprinkle toasted almonds on salads, granola, cereal and steamed vegetables; spread almond butter on a sandwich or toast; and crush almonds to use as a coating on chicken or fish. Want an even greater nutrient kick? Mix almonds with dried apricots and fortified whole-grain cereal for a fresh trail mix. (Just watch the portion size because calories can add up quickly.)

2. KALE | **SERVING SIZE: ½ CUP COOKED** Spinach gets more attention, but kale is a great alternative because spinach contains oxalate, a compound that inhibits calcium absorption. "Kale is low in calories but high in vitamins A and C, both of which help with wound healing (important if you've had a Cesarean section or episiotomy) and recovery from childbirth," says Tubman.
TIPS To prepare kale, boil it for a minute or two, then sauté it as you would spinach or any other leafy green; the initial blanching will soften the texture. Add it to salads, soups, pasta dishes or casseroles; or mix it into mashed potatoes.

Prenatals postpartum?

Should you continue taking your prenatal vitamins while you're breastfeeing? That depends, says Melinda Johnson, M.S., R.D. If you're eating a healthy balanced diet, it may not be necessary; however, new mothers should at least take 400 micrograms of folic acid daily because they could become pregnant again, Johnson says. (This B vitamin helps prevent neural-tube defects, such as spina bifida.) Some doctors prefer that all breastfeeding women continue taking their prenatal vitamins.

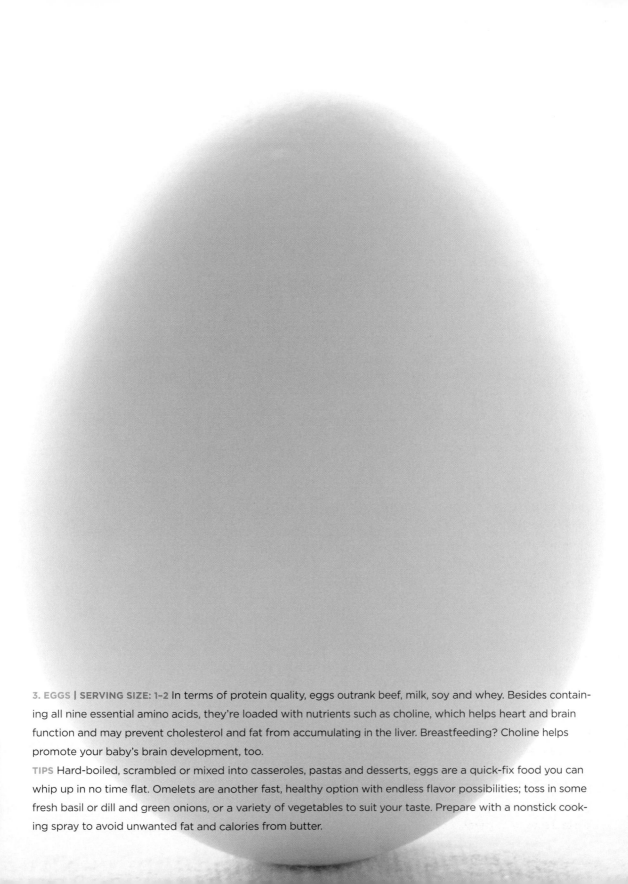

3. EGGS | **SERVING SIZE: 1–2** In terms of protein quality, eggs outrank beef, milk, soy and whey. Besides containing all nine essential amino acids, they're loaded with nutrients such as choline, which helps heart and brain function and may prevent cholesterol and fat from accumulating in the liver. Breastfeeding? Choline helps promote your baby's brain development, too.

TIPS Hard-boiled, scrambled or mixed into casseroles, pastas and desserts, eggs are a quick-fix food you can whip up in no time flat. Omelets are another fast, healthy option with endless flavor possibilities; toss in some fresh basil or dill and green onions, or a variety of vegetables to suit your taste. Prepare with a nonstick cooking spray to avoid unwanted fat and calories from butter.

4. SALMON | **SERVING SIZE: 3 OZ., UP TO 12 OZ. PER WEEK** Salmon is low in mercury and high in omega-3 fatty acids, particularly DHA, a nutrient that's crucial for the development of your baby's brain and nervous system. It also helps prevent postpartum depression and enhance immune function. "Pay attention to the DHA in your diet when you're nursing," says Johnson. "If you don't get enough of it, your body will rob your stores."
TIPS Eat salmon broiled, baked or lightly pan-fried with a heart-healthy oil, such as olive oil. Choose wild salmon because it contains more omega-3s and fewer pollutants than farmed salmon.

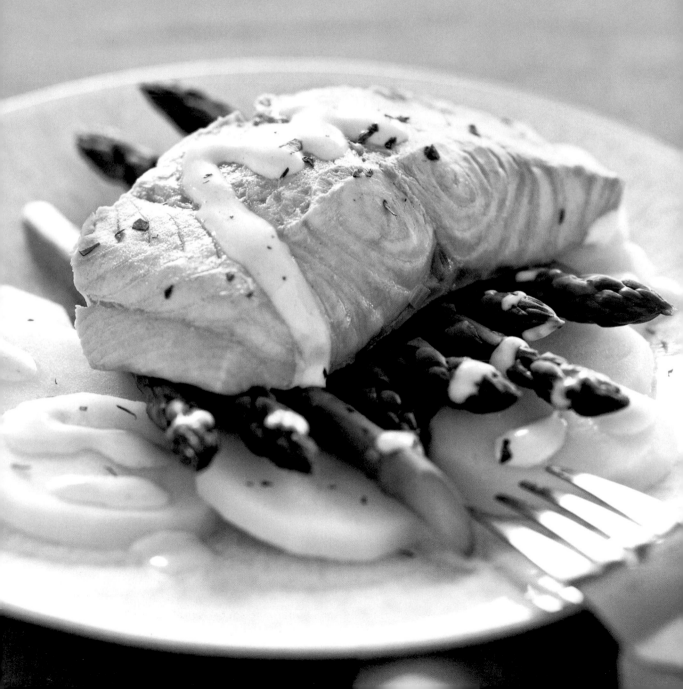

✳ Salmon is good for your baby's brainpower and your own mood.

5. LENTILS | SERVING SIZE: 1/2 CUP Lentils are easy to prepare, high in fiber and one of the best sources of iron. "Because of blood loss during and after delivery, you may have lost a lot of iron," says Johnson. "Low iron can translate to low energy, but you can get it back by eating foods that are iron-rich." Concerned about getting rid of those extra pregnancy pounds? The fiber in lentils can help you feel full without a lot of extra calories. Lentils are also a good source of folate, which may be low if you've stopped taking your prenatal vitamins. (See "Prenatals Postpartum?," pg. 50.)

TIPS Toss cooked lentils into soups, salads and pasta recipes; mix them with rice, quinoa or other grains; or use them as a base for bean dip. You can also mix cooked lentils into brownie batter for an extra fiber boost; you won't be able to taste them, but you'll get the nutritional benefits while satisfying your sweet tooth.

6. YOGURT | SERVING SIZE: 1 CUP Yogurt is more nutrient-dense than milk, boasting higher concentrations of protein, calcium and vitamin D. It's great for new moms because protein is necessary for muscle and tissue repair and rebuilding after childbirth. "And, it's a good source of zinc, which is another healing nutrient," says Tubman. Protein from your breast milk also helps provide building blocks for your baby's growth. Yogurt contains live, active bacterial cultures that can aid digestion and help alleviate gastrointestinal distress, but some brands undergo heat processing that kills these beneficial bacteria. Look for brands bearing the National Yogurt Association's Live & Active Cultures seal; this signifies that they contain at least 100 million cultures per gram of yogurt, the amount deemed appropriate for health benefits.

TIPS In addition to snacking on fruit and yogurt to power through your morning, try incorporating yogurt into savory sauces as an alternative to sour cream. Also mix it into thicker soups, such as black bean or pumpkin.

Naughty foods made nice

You can still have your favorite comfort foods and eat them, too. The following recipes make use of a few clever culinary swaps that are so flavorful you won't even wonder where the fat went. And, you'll also get essential nutrients without feeling deprived.

CHEESEBURGER WITH SWEET POTATO OVEN FRIES
Serves 6

Prep time: fries, 15 minutes
burgers, 20 minutes
Cooking time: fries, 50 minutes
burgers, 7 minutes

For fries
1½ pounds sweet potatoes (about 3 small)
1 tablespoon olive oil
½ teaspoon paprika
Salt and freshly ground black pepper, to taste

For burgers
6 whole-grain buns
3 cloves garlic
1 7-ounce box button mushrooms, cleaned
½ pound lean ground turkey
¼ pound lean ground beef
1 large egg
2 teaspoons Dijon mustard
1 teaspoon Worcestershire sauce
¼ teaspoon coarse salt
¼ teaspoon ground black pepper
2½ teaspoons olive oil
6 slices reduced-fat Cheddar cheese
6 whole-wheat hamburger buns

To make fries: Preheat oven to 400° F. Coat a baking sheet with nonstick cooking spray. Cut sweet potatoes into spears. Place in a large bowl, add oil and paprika, then transfer to baking sheet. Bake for 50 minutes, turning potatoes three times during cooking so they brown evenly. Season with salt and pepper to taste.

To make burgers: Tear bread into pieces and place in a food processor. Process into fine crumbs, then transfer crumbs to a large bowl. Add garlic and mince. Add mushrooms and process until ground. Transfer mixture to bowl with crumbs. Add ground turkey, beef, egg, mustard, Worcestershire, salt and pepper. Mix until well blended. Shape meat into six patties.

Heat olive oil in a large nonstick skillet over medium-high heat. Add burgers and cook for 5 minutes on each side, or until cooked through. Place cheese over each burger, cover pan, cook over low heat until cheese is melted and serve on a whole-wheat bun.

[Per serving] **(1 burger plus 4 oz. fries): 460 calories, 46% carbohydrate (53 g), 30% fat (16 g), 24% protein (28 g), 7 g fiber, 221 mg calcium, 4 mg iron, 4 mg vitamin C, 93 mcg folate.**

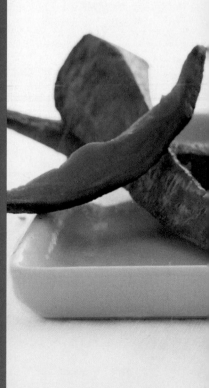

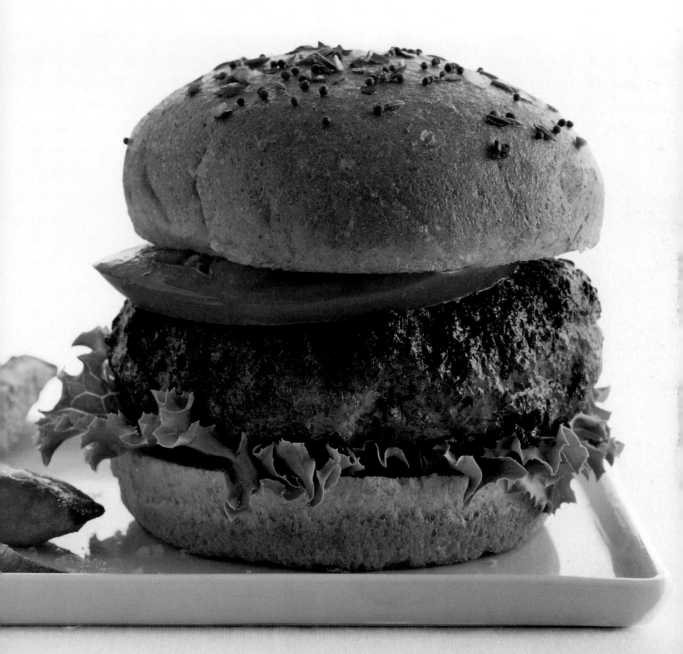

**Cheeseburger with Sweet
Potato Oven Fries**

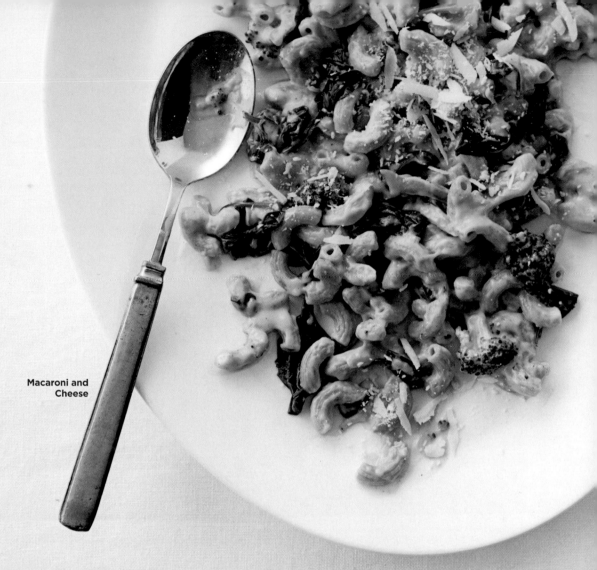

Macaroni and Cheese

MACARONI AND CHEESE
Serves 6

Prep time: 10 minutes
Cooking time: 15 minutes

1 ³/₄ cups fat-free evaporated
        milk, divided
3   tablespoons flour
1   teaspoon Dijon mustard
½   teaspoon garlic powder
½   teaspoon paprika
½   teaspoon coarse salt
¼   teaspoon ground nutmeg
4   ounces shredded reduced-fat
        sharp Cheddar cheese
        (about 1 cup)
³/₄ pound whole-wheat
        macaroni
1   10-ounce package frozen
        chopped broccoli
6   cups baby spinach leaves,
        rinsed
6   tablespoons grated Pecorino
        Romano cheese

Place a large pot of water over
high heat for boiling pasta. Place 1
cup of evaporated milk in a large
saucepan. Pour remaining ³/₄ cup
into a medium bowl and whisk
in flour, mustard, garlic powder,
paprika, salt and nutmeg.

Bring evaporated milk to a
simmer over medium heat. Whisk
in flour mixture and cook, whisk-
ing constantly, until mixture has
thickened, about 2 to 3 minutes.
Remove from heat and whisk in
Cheddar cheese until melted.

Cover to keep warm.

Cook broccoli according to
package directions, then drain.
Add pasta to boiling water and
cook 6 minutes. Add spinach and
cook 30 seconds more, just until
wilted. Drain pasta and spinach
and blend into cheese sauce,
along with broccoli. Stir pasta
and cheese over medium-low
heat until mixture is hot, about
1 minute. Top each serving with
1 tablespoon of Pecorino
Romano cheese.

[Per serving] (1 cup): 360 calories,
62% carbohydrate (56 g), 22% protein
(20 g), 16% fat (7 g), 7 g fiber, 545 mg
calcium, 28 mg vitamin C, 3 mg iron,
125 mcg folate.

SPICED CARROT CUPCAKES
Serves 12

Prep time: 40 minutes
Cooking time: 30 minutes

For cupcakes
½ cup unsweetened canned pumpkin purée
1 8-ounce can crushed pineapple, drained
1 cup shredded carrots
½ cup golden raisins
¾ cup granulated sugar
1 large egg
1 large egg white
¼ cup canola oil
1⅓ cups whole-wheat pastry flour
1 teaspoon baking powder
1½ teaspoons pumpkin pie spice
½ teaspoon baking soda
½ teaspoon coarse salt
¼ cup chopped walnuts

For frosting
6 ounces reduced-fat cream cheese
¾ cup confectioners' sugar
1 teaspoon vanilla extract
2 tablespoons chopped candied ginger

To make cupcakes: Preheat oven to 350° F. Place cupcake wrappers in muffin pan. Place pumpkin purée in a large bowl with pineapple, carrots and raisins. Stir to blend. Add sugar, egg, egg white and oil and stir until well mixed.

In a medium bowl, whisk together flour, pumpkin pie spice, baking powder, baking soda and salt. Add to wet ingredients, add walnuts and stir until blended.

Spoon batter into cupcake cups and bake for 30 minutes. Let cupcakes cool in pan, then transfer to a plate.

To make frosting: Combine cream cheese, sugar and vanilla in a medium bowl. With a mixer, blend until smooth. Frost cupcakes and garnish with candied ginger.

[Per serving] (1 cupcake): 272 calories, 59% carbohydrate (40 g), 32% fat (10 g), 9% protein (6 g), 3 g fiber, 62 mg calcium, 3 mg vitamin C, 1 mg iron, 15 mcg folate.

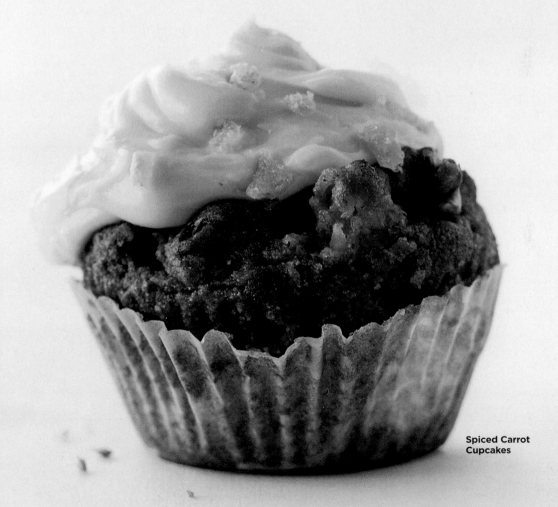

Spiced Carrot Cupcakes

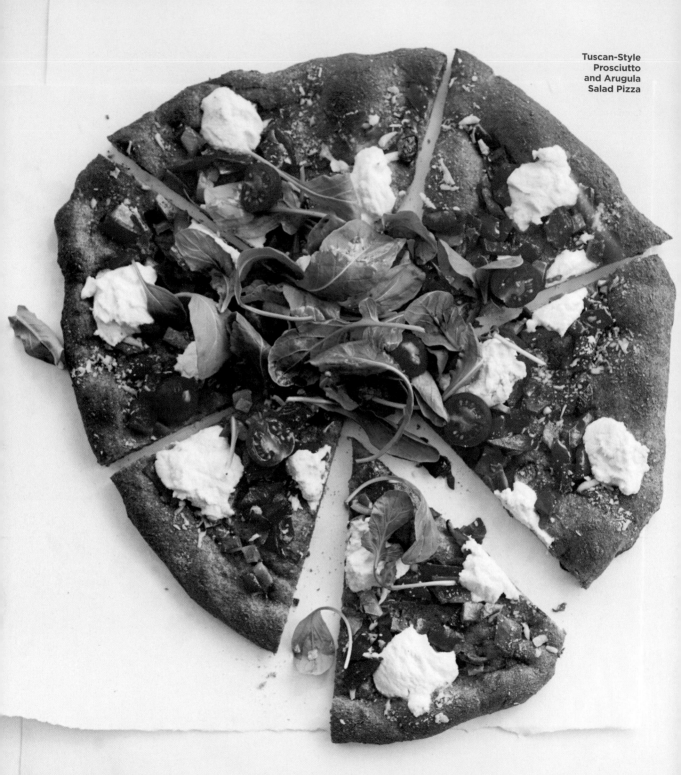

Tuscan-Style Prosciutto and Arugula Salad Pizza

A typical pepperoni pizza is loaded with saturated fat. This slimmed-down version offers vitamin C, iron, fiber and folate.

TUSCAN-STYLE PROSCIUTTO AND ARUGULA SALAD PIZZA
Serves 6
Prep time: 25 minutes
Cooking time: 20 minutes

1 12-ounce package prepared whole-wheat pizza dough
Cornmeal and flour for sprinkling
4 teaspoons olive oil
1 large red onion, peeled and chopped
1 sweet red pepper, cored, seeded and chopped
3 ounces sliced prosciutto, cut into bite-size pieces
Salt and freshly ground black pepper
2 ounces grated Pecorino Romano cheese (about ½ cup)
1 cup low-fat ricotta cheese
3 cups baby arugula leaves, rinsed
1 pint cherry tomatoes, each cut in half
1 teaspoon balsamic vinegar

Place a cold pizza stone (or inverted baking sheet) on middle oven rack and preheat oven to 500° F, at least 20 minutes. Generously sprinkle a wooden pizza peel or the back of another baking sheet with cornmeal.

Meanwhile, heat 2 teaspoons olive oil in a large nonstick skillet over medium-high heat. Add peeled and chopped onion, cored, seeded and chopped pepper and sliced prosciutto and sauté 12 minutes, or until onion is golden and prosciutto starts to get crisp.

Sprinkle a clean work surface with flour. Roll out the prepared whole-wheat dough to form a 13-inch circle. Transfer to prepared wooden pizza peel (or back of baking sheet). Slide dough circle onto heated pizza stone or baking sheet and cook for 5 minutes; remove from oven.

Scatter onion-prosciutto mixture evenly over dough and sprinkle with Pecorino Romano cheese. Drop dabs of low-fat ricotta cheese over entire pizza and bake again for 12 to 15 minutes, or until edges are golden and underside of crust, when lifted up, is browned.

While pizza cooks, place arugula and tomato halves in a salad bowl. Add remaining olive oil and balsamic vinegar. Season with salt and pepper and toss. Cut pizza into 6 slices. Scatter salad over pizza and serve.

[Per serving] (1 slice): 314 calories, 44% carbohydrate (35 g), 34% fat (12 g), 22% protein (18 g), 7 g fiber, 298 mg calcium, 56 mg vitamin C, 1.9 mg iron, 102 mcg folate.

Naughty & nice swaps

Oversized cheeseburgers and greasy pizza may be two of your favorite indulgences, but they can hamper your nutrition goals. Try these healthy alternatives instead:

Instead of ...	Try ...
Bakery pastry	Whole-wheat frozen waffle topped with low-fat cream cheese and all-fruit preserves
Fast-food cheeseburger	Black-bean burger with reduced-fat cheese on a whole-wheat bun
Ice cream milkshake	Low-fat frozen yogurt
Potato chips	Reduced-sodium baked potato chips
Scrambled eggs with sausage	Scrambled eggs with chopped bell peppers and low-fat chicken sausage
Grilled cheese sandwich on white bread	Whole-grain bread with reduced-fat cheese grilled in a skillet with nonstick cooking spray

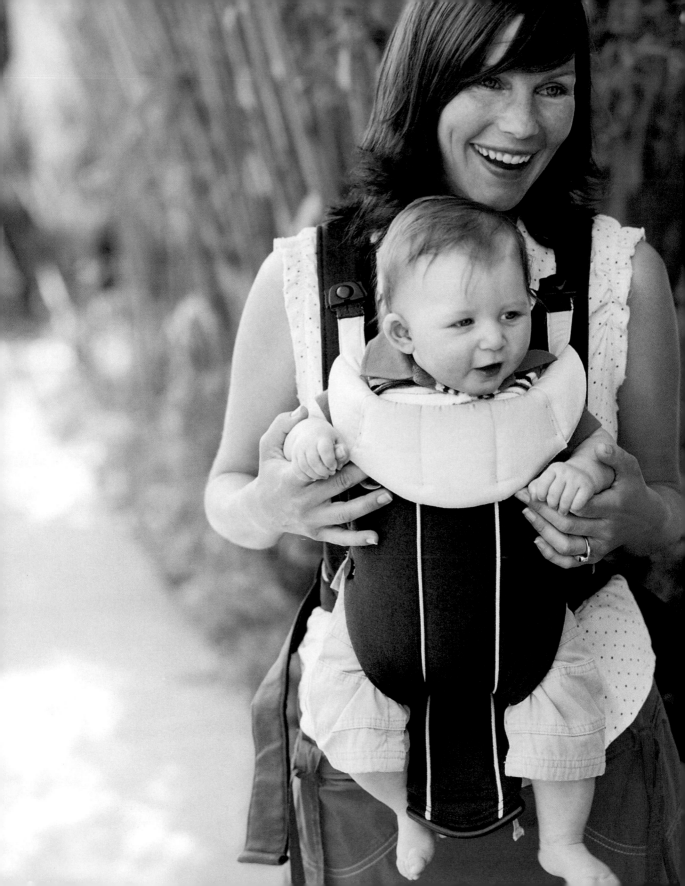

EXERCISE AFTER BABY | 3

Exercise is the key to getting your pre-baby

body back. Not only do regular workouts strengthen and tone your muscles, they also help contribute to weight loss and boost your mood. The sooner you start moving, the better: Research shows that the first six months after childbirth are critical to losing the baby weight—and keeping it off.

Getting started is as easy as taking a walk around the block. The following 12-month walking plan will gradually build your stamina and strength. When you're ready for more, move on to the whole-body conditioning workouts or zone in on your trouble areas with targeted core and abdominal moves. Need some extra motivation? Plan a workout with other moms. Walking or hiking with other new parents is a fun way to get your exercise—and a means to feeling connected and combating the isolation of being a new mother.

For each workout, follow the suggested guidelines for safety. Wait at least six weeks before starting select workouts; longer if you've had a Cesarean section. You should also check with your doctor before beginning any exercise program.

For most women, once pregnancy is over, you're suddenly in unfamiliar territory: Welcome to Postpartumville! Here, objects in the mirror were once smaller than they appear and the roadblocks can be bumpy, flabby and, most of all, saggy. Not to worry: There are expert territory surveyors—doctors, trainers, and physical therapists—who can help guide you, body part by body part, through this strange new land.

Upper body

THE PROBLEM Many moms-to-be don't stick to a regular upper-body workout during pregnancy, leading to flabbiness and weakness. Additionally, your body produces the hormone relaxin, which loosens the joints, in larger amounts during pregnancy; this can weaken the joints afterward. As a result, out-of-shape arms are ill-equipped to lift a baby from car seat to crib to stroller to changing table and back again several times a day, while wrists and shoulders may hurt and feel weak.

THE SOLUTION Toning and strengthening the arms, back and shoulder muscles can also help relieve strain on the wrists. The best time to start is during pregnancy, says Megan Flatt, a trainer and fitness educator in San Francisco and creator of Bump Fitness, a program of prenatal and post-baby fitness workouts. After giving birth, wait six weeks before starting to exercise, says Flatt.

Swollen fingers and ankles

THE PROBLEM "During pregnancy your body produces roughly 50 percent more blood and other fluids than normal to accommodate your growing baby," says Lyssie Lakatos, R.D., C.D.N., C.F.T., a personal trainer and nutritionist in New York. Hormone fluctuations can also contribute to edema, or swelling of the hands, face, ankles, neck and other extremities. It can take weeks for all the extra fluids to leave your system.

THE SOLUTION "Choose foods rich in potassium, such as fruits and vegetables; it helps counteract the water-retaining effects of sodium [salt]," says Lakatos who also recommends drinking more than the recommended eight glasses of water per day, especially if you are nursing.

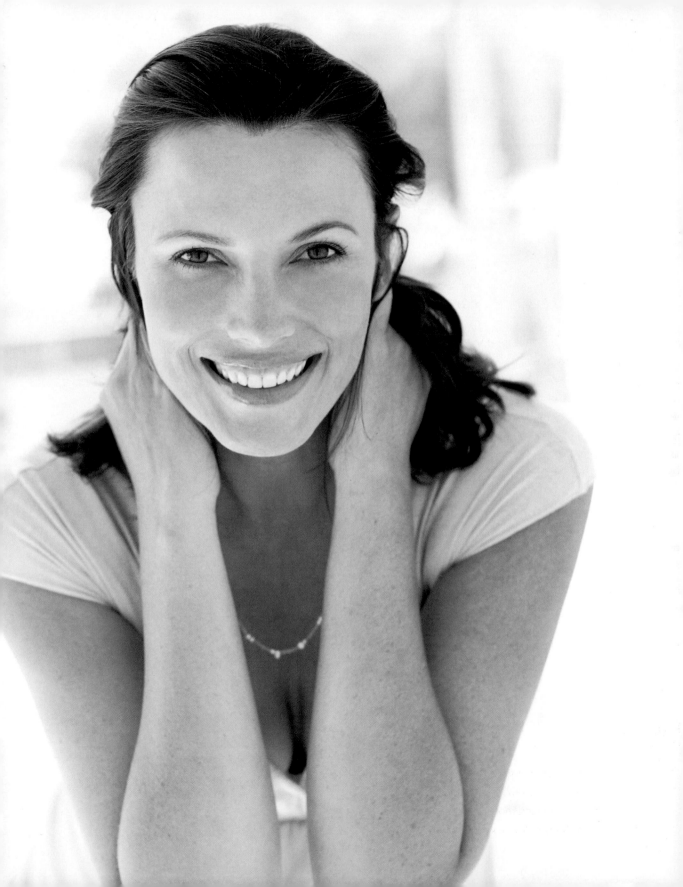

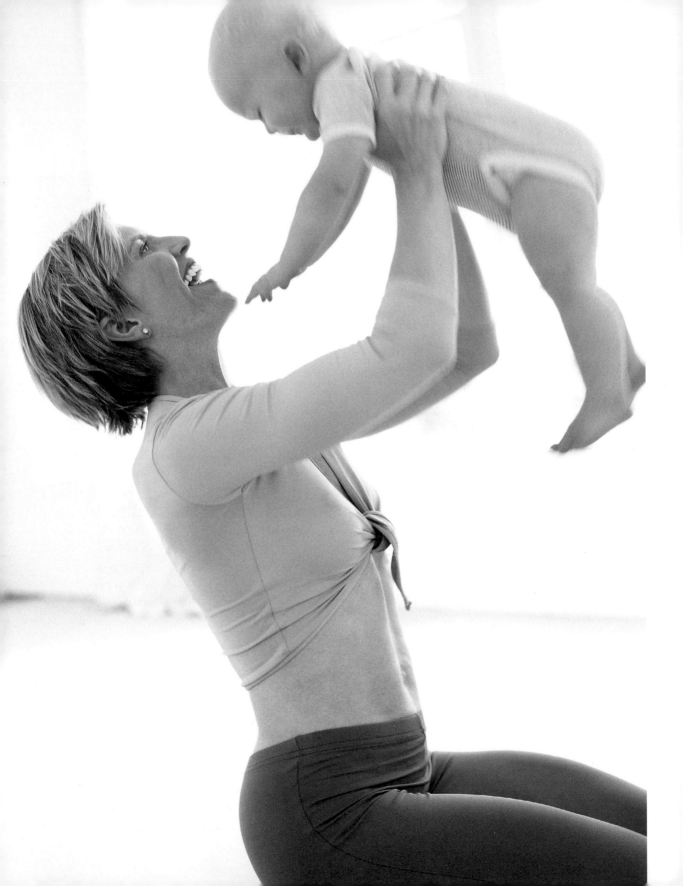

Breasts

THE PROBLEM Immediately after delivery, your breasts become larger as they fill first with colostrum and then with milk; most will stay that size for a few weeks. Breastfeeding mothers will experience enlarged breasts for as long as they nurse exclusively. The whole process, including being pregnant, causes most women's breast tissue to stretch, whether they breastfeed or not. "Once pregnancy and nursing end, most women lose breast volume, retain stretch marks and experience some sagging," says Robert Brueck, M.D., a Fort Myers, Fla.-based board-certified plastic surgeon with 30 years of experience in mommy makeovers: a package of cosmetic surgery procedures that includes a tummy tuck, breast work and liposuction. The nipple may also look displaced.

THE SOLUTION Most women accept the changes in their breasts as a rite of passage to motherhood. Some may want to do exercises to firm up the chest wall behind the breasts, "lifting" them a bit. But depending on a woman's level of discomfort with how her breasts look, the most satisfactory solution may be surgery.

Belly

THE PROBLEM Your belly undergoes more changes during pregnancy than any other body part. Depending on your age, genetics and the amount of weight you gain, this can mean stretch marks and excess flab, or a "pooch," postpartum. It can take as long as six weeks for the uterus to revert back to its old size, which will decrease the size of your belly. But since the abdominal skin has been stretched and pulled, it may never again be as taut as it was. Additionally, some women will be left with stretch marks (these are largely hereditary).

THE SOLUTION "Keeping the core muscles [abdominals and back] strong during pregnancy helps the abdominals recover faster," says Flatt. As for that extra pooch, most experts recommend Pilates-based abdominal work. A balanced diet, along with regular workouts that include targeted abdominal exercise will get most women the results they want. (For abdominal workouts, see pgs. 82-87.) If working out doesn't do this for you, a tummy tuck will.

*When you're expecting, your belly undergoes more changes than any other body part.

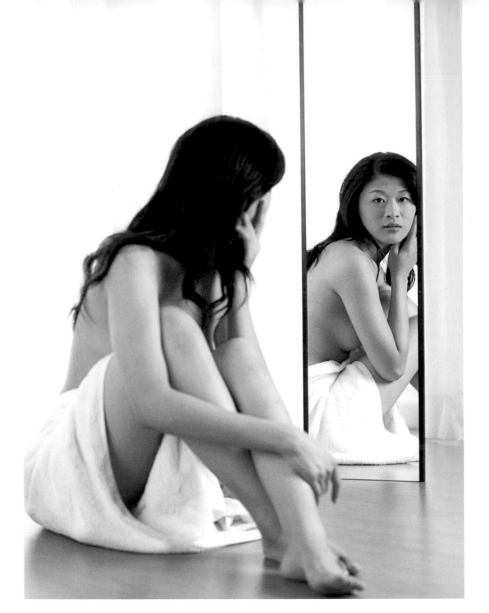

Thighs, hips, buttocks

THE PROBLEM "During pregnancy, very often a woman's activity and nutrition levels go down," says OB-GYN Michael Dawson, M.D., a member of Atlanta Women's Specialists. "These factors mean you gain weight. The extra fat then gets distributed to places where women most often put on weight: the backside, hips and thighs." Even if you do continue your healthy eating and exercise routine, pregnancy alone may determine where you put on extra pounds.

THE SOLUTION It can take up to a year to lose the weight gained during pregnancy, says Dawson. To shed pounds gradually, experts recommend a mix of exercise and well-balanced nutrition. Low-calorie, high-fiber foods, such as vegetables, promote a feeling of fullness, making it easier to eat less. As for exercise, Flatt recommends moves that work multiple muscles. (For full-body workouts that will strengthen those muscles you use most as a new mom, see "Moves That Multi-Task," pgs. 74-77, and "Moves For Mothers," pgs. 78-79.)

Vaginal region

THE PROBLEM Women who had a vaginal delivery often experience tearing of the perineum (the area between the vaginal opening and anus) or had an episiotomy (a surgical incision through the perineum), both of which need at least six weeks to heal. Incontinence, or the inability to stop urine from leaking, is also a common complaint. Some women also experience painful intercourse or pelvic organ prolapse, a condition in which the bladder, uterus or rectum falls out of its normal position, straining the pelvic-floor muscles.

THE SOLUTION Kegels, Kegels, Kegels, says Suzanne Aceron Badillo, P.T., W.S.C., clinical program director of the Women's Health Rehabilitation Program at the Rehabilitation Institute of Chicago. By tightening and then releasing the muscles surrounding the vagina, Kegels strengthen the pelvic floor. This helps control bladder function and stabilizes the pelvic area. (For more exercises targeting the pelvic floor, see pgs. 108-109.) In cases of painful intercourse, relaxation is key. If you've had an incision or tear in the perineum, you may be unconsciously flexing your pelvic floor, which can cause sex to hurt, says Badillo. To help prevent a tear in the perineum, Badillo suggests performing a daily massage of the area in the final weeks of pregnancy. Postpartum, a daily massage will help a scar become more pliant.

> * Kegels strengthen the pelvic floor, which helps control bladder function and stabilizes the pelvic area.

Feet

THE PROBLEM When you're expecting, your extra weight, shifting center of gravity and swelling can often increase your foot size (usually by a half size) and sometimes permanently. "During pregnancy, there is a slight tilt of the body forward," says Philadelphia podiatrist Edward Chairman, D.P.M. "Because nature wants to compensate, the forefoot spreads and the arch flattens, causing the foot size to increase." Additionally, the extra weight of pregnancy puts pressure on the veins in the legs, causing your feet to swell.

THE SOLUTION Chairman recommends being fit for an orthotic (a device worn inside the shoe that can help correct posture) and, for best results, to do so early in your pregnancy. Post-pregnancy, an orthotic can help prevent further damage. And, of course, whenever posible, Chairman encourages moms to "sit down and put their feet up."

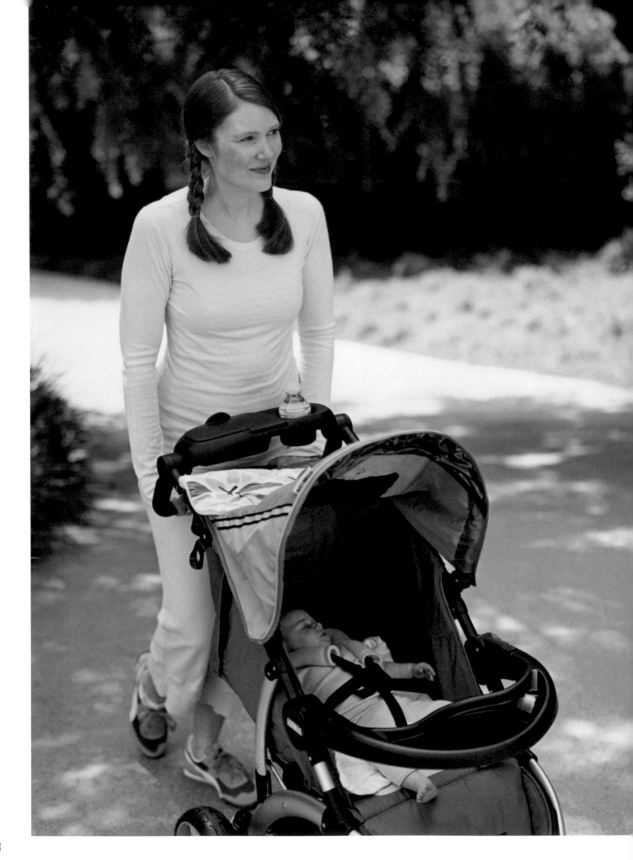

Best baby weight busters

Many new moms find exercise the key to losing the baby weight, and studies support their experience. A 2007 Harvard University study of new moms found that women who walked 30 minutes each day had a 34 percent lower chance of retaining a significant amount of weight (defined as 11 pounds or more) at their baby's first birthday. Research also shows that exercise helps new moms preserve muscle mass—and thus appear more toned—than moms who drop weight just by dieting.

Combine nutrition with exercise

Weight loss also hinges on smart food choices. In a study funded by the National Institutes of Health, Cheryl A. Lovelady, Ph.D., R.D., a nutrition professor at the University of North Carolina at Greensboro, followed 40 overweight breastfeeding moms starting at one month postpartum. One group achieved a 500-calorie-a-day deficit by following a nutritious diet and doing moderate exercise, primarily walking. The other moms didn't modify their eating habits or exercise. After four months, the diet-and-exercise group had lost 10 pounds; the other group had lost only 1 pound on average, and some had actually gained weight. "The first six months are critical," says Lovelady, who notes that while you can lose the baby weight after six months, your risk for obesity is higher the longer you wait. Exercise has other advantages, says Lovelady, such as strengthening the heart and helping prevent type II diabetes.

Calorie counter

activity	calories/hour
walking	316
yoga	243
Pilates	226
strength training	210

NOTE: CALORIE BURN IS BASED ON A 135-POUND WOMAN.

 Research shows that regular exercise helps new moms preserve muscle mass and thus appear more toned.

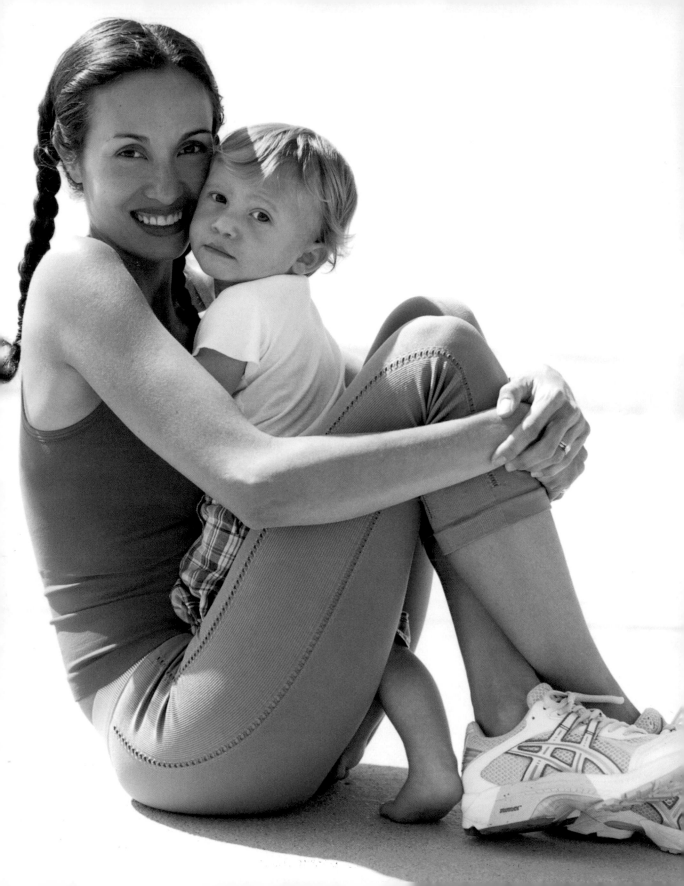

Walk it off

After having a baby, walking is one of the best ways to start moving your body—and shed the pounds gained during pregnancy. The following 12-month walk/jog program is designed to build energy and stamina. Overall, be patient. Many women find that it takes a year to really start feeling—and looking—like themselves again.

MONTH 1 | Until you get your doctor's OK to resume working out (usually at your six-week checkup, later if you had a Cesarean section), don't do anything more strenuous than taking easy walks; use this time to get a feel for your body again. Try to get out every day, even if it's for only 10 minutes or so—put your baby in a front carrier or stroller and take him with you. (If walking causes or makes any bleeding worse, stop immediately and contact your doctor.)

MONTH 2 | Now is the time to start building your stamina. Gradually increase the length of your walks until you're at approximately 100 minutes total per week. Make it a habit:Try to walk at least five days a week.

MONTH 3 | Keep walking five days a week, increasing your total time to about 150 minutes. Add a few speed bursts to your walks. (To do a speed burst, pick up the pace for about a minute, then resume your normal pace for one minute.)

MONTH 4 | Increase the length of your speed bursts so you're doing a burst of three minutes, followed by one minute at your normal pace; complete four bursts each time you walk. Try to walk six days a week, totaling 180 minutes.

MONTH 5 | Increase your total walking time to 200 minutes per week, making sure at least one walk is 45 minutes long. Increase your speed bursts to about four minutes each; do five of them each time you walk.

MONTH 6 | Take it up a notch by going for some easy climbing on gentle hills one day a week. (If you are walking with your baby, for comfort and safety, it may be time to move him to a sturdy backpack or jogging stroller.) Continue to

* Move it to lose it: Walking is one of the best ways to shed the baby weight.

71

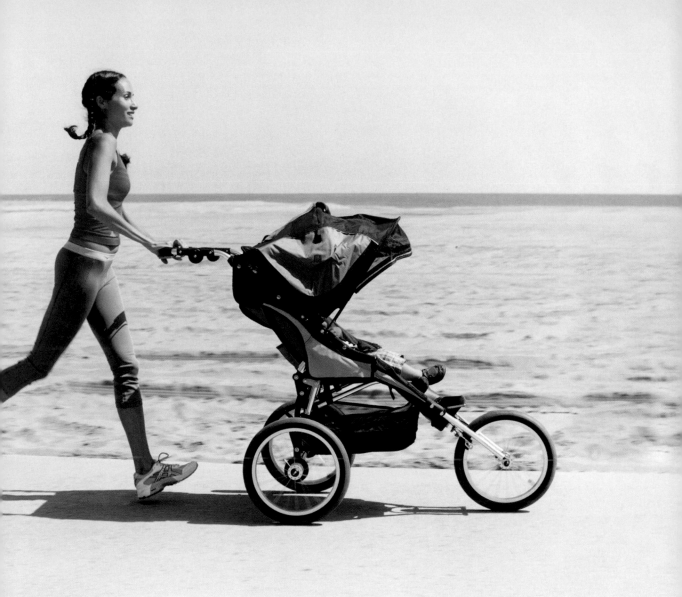

* Most new moms can begin a gentle walking program at about six weeks after delivery. You can use a front carrier or stroller so your baby can come with you.

walk six days a week, for a total of 210 minutes. (Climbing takes the place of speed bursts this month and the following month, too.)

MONTH 7 | Add another day of climbing gentle hills to your routine. Continue to walk six days a week, for a total of 200 minutes. (The extra time spent on hills compensates for the fewer total minutes this month.)

MONTH 8 | Now it's time to add speed bursts back into your routine. Walk six days a week, for a total of 225 minutes. Aim to do six five-minute speed bursts on five days and 50 minutes of hiking another day.

MONTH 9 | Add a bit of jogging to your workouts to challenge your body with both greater impact and a faster pace. (If you are walking/jogging with your baby, move him to a jogging stroller if you haven't already done so.) Exercise six days a week: Do your normal walking routine for four days; on two days, add four one-minute intervals of jogging, followed by one minute of walking. Total jogging time: eight minutes a week. Total exercise time: 216 minutes.

MONTH 10 | Aim to get in at least one long walk every week that lasts approximately 60 minutes. Continue to exercise six days a week, and build in even more jogging. Include two days in which you jog for two minutes and walk for one; do four intervals. Total jogging time: 16 minutes a week. Total exercise time: 230 minutes.

MONTH 11 | Increase your jogging time to 15 minutes twice a week (jog for 15 minutes straight or do jog/walk intervals). Continue to exercise six days a week. Total jogging time: 30 minutes a week. Total exercise time: 230 minutes.

MONTH 12 | Continue to exercise six days a week while increasing your jogging time. Total jogging time: 40 minutes a week. Total exercise time: 230 minutes.

Energy booster

Moms who suffer from postpartum depression may feel even more tired than other rookie mothers, says Maria Dritsa, Ph.D., the author of a study on postpartum fatigue conducted at McGill University in Montreal. Surprisingly, treatment for this symptom of new motherhood may include regular workouts.

When Dritsa looked at depressed moms four to 38 weeks after delivery, she found that those who followed an at-home exercise program were significantly less fatigued, both physically and mentally. The exercisers averaged a bit more than two hours weekly of aerobic exercise, such as brisk walking or jogging.

Drista recommends that new moms stay alert to the signs of exhaustion and consult their doctor if the symptoms continue.

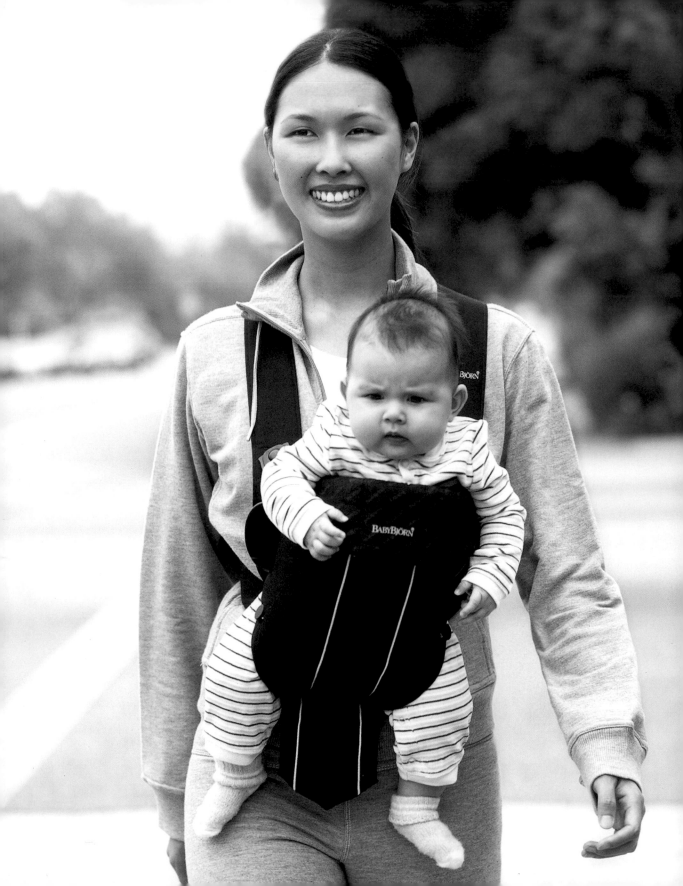

Moves that multi-task
Build all-over strength with four
exercises that work multiple muscles.

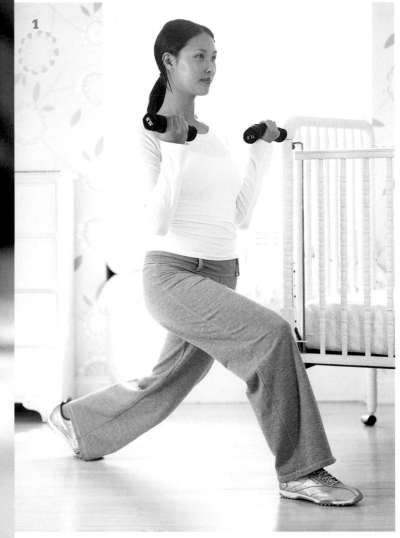

The following workout, which was designed by Patrea Aeschliman, owner of Go Mom Fitness in Indianapolis, is an at-home strength-training program that will recondition and strengthen your body. Plus, these time-saving moves work multiple muscles simultaneously, which helps speed metabolism and burns more calories, says Aeschliman. With your doctor's OK, begin doing this workout one to two days per week, gradually increasing the number of days as you get stronger. Do one set of 10–15 repetitions for each exercise in the given order, resting 30 seconds between moves. Begin by doing these moves without weights, then try using 3- to 5-pound dumbbells. When you feel strong enough, add the bonus move to each repetition.

 Warm up
If possible, take a 10- to 15-minute walk to warm up your muscles, or dance to get your heart rate up a bit. Then roll your shoulders forward and back, and do wrist and ankle rolls clockwise, then counter-clockwise, 5 times each way.

1 WALKING LUNGE WITH CURL Stand with your arms at your sides, holding dumbbells, feet hip-width apart. Keeping shoulders relaxed and abs drawn in, take a big step forward with your right leg, bending both knees 90 degrees. Keep right knee over right ankle, left knee approaching the floor but not touching. Bend elbows, curling the weights toward shoulders [shown]. Straighten arms, then push off your back foot to the starting position. (1 rep equals 1 lunge on each side).
Bonus move: Do a knee lift before you step forward.

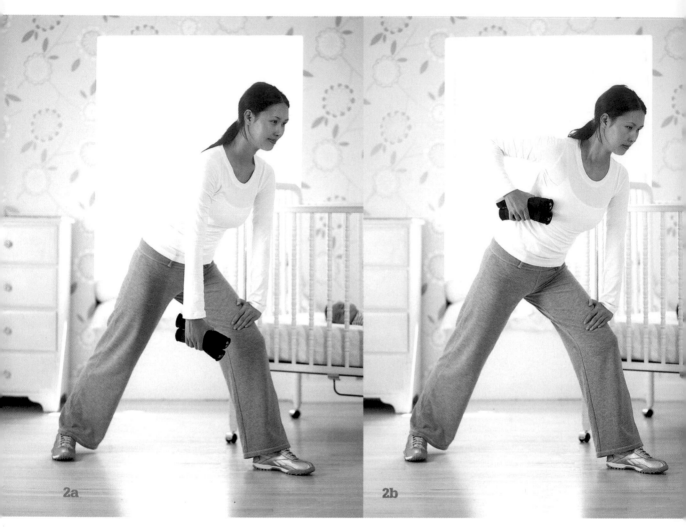

2a

2b

2 **SIDE LUNGE WITH ROW** Holding two dumbbells in your right hand, stand with feet hip-width apart, abs and pelvic-floor muscles drawn in. Take a big step to the left, bending the knee, left hand on thigh for support, right arm hanging straight down. Keep your right leg straight and your foot flat **[A]**. Bend your right elbow, bringing the weight to your upper ribs **[B]**. Lower the weight and push off on your left foot to starting position. Complete reps then switch sides.
Bonus move: Bend your knee deeper and touch your front ankle at the bottom of the lunge.

3 BRIDGE AND PRESS

Lie on your back, holding a dumbbell in each hand. Bend your knees and rest your feet flat on the floor, keeping your abs and pelvic-floor muscles drawn in. Bend your elbows and place your upper arms on the floor, your forearms vertical and parallel to each other. Straighten your arms, pressing the weights up in front of your chest [A]. Bend your elbows and lower the weights, then, with your knees bent, lift your hips, pressing your heels into the floor until your body forms one straight line from your head to your hips [B]. Lower your hips and complete reps.
Bonus move: Hold your hips up in this "bridge" while you do the press.

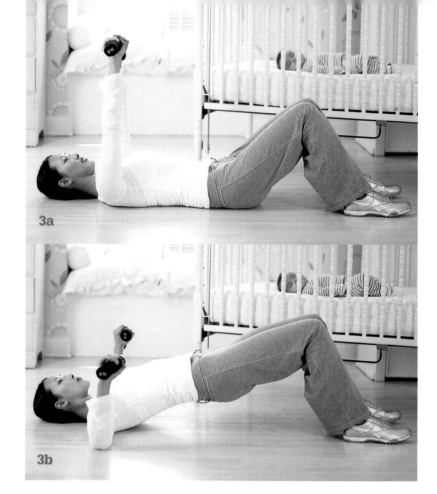

3a

3b

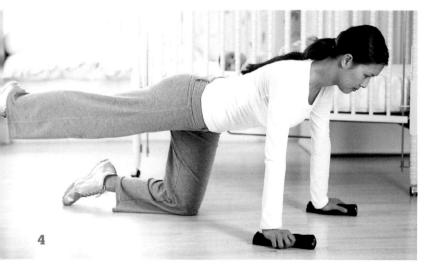

4

4 LEG LIFT WITH KNEE PULL

Kneel on all fours with a weight in each hand, hands wider than your shoulders, your knees under your hip. Keeping your abs drawn in and your neck long, lift your right leg out behind you at hip height, squeezing your buttocks [shown]. Pull your right knee in toward your chest and draw in your abs. Lift your leg back to hip height and complete reps. Switch legs, repeat.
Bonus move: As you lift your leg to hip height, bend your elbows and do a push-up.

✳ Cool down
Stretch your legs, hips, chest and arms, holding each stretch for 30 seconds without bouncing. Be sure to breathe deeply; in through your nose and out through your mouth, drawing your belly in.

Moves for mothers
Four exercises that target the muscles you use most as a new mom.

As a new mom, you're likely lifting your baby from crib to changing table to car seat to stroller (and back again!) several times each day. The following four exercises are designed to strengthen and tone the muscles you use most, including your legs, back and shoulders. Start with two days a week and add a day or two when you're ready.

When exercising, be sure to follow these safety tips: Keep your abdominals and pelvic-floor muscles drawn in; inhale deeply through your nose and exhale through your mouth; when using dumbbells, do not grip them too tightly; and, drink plenty of water before, during and after your workout.

Wait at least six weeks before beginning this workout. Always get your doctor's OK before starting this or any exercise program.

1

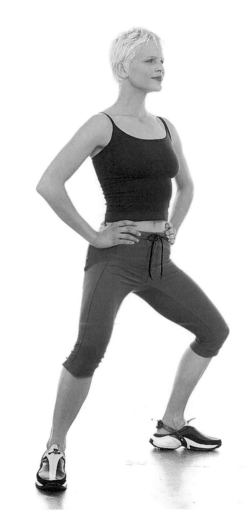

1 **EASY PLIÉ** Stand with feet farther than shoulder-width apart, toes and knees turned out, hands on hips. Keep torso erect, abs pulled in and heels on the floor as you slowly bend your knees and lower your torso without tilting your pelvis forward or back [shown]. Make sure your knees don't extend beyond your toes. Rise slowly to starting position; repeat. Do 2–3 sets of 15 reps.

2

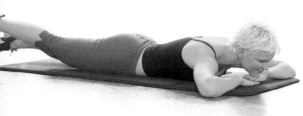

2 FLUTTER KICK Lie facedown on the floor with your legs straight and toes pointed, elbows bent, hands in front of your face. Rest your chin on your hands, eyes focused downward, and lift your abs away from the floor. Without bending the knee, slowly lift your right leg about 4 inches off the floor. Bring your right leg down as you raise your left leg, keeping hips stationary and in contact with the floor [shown]. Continue to alternate for 25–50 reps.

3 PUSH-UP Kneel on all fours, arms straight and knees under hips, hip-width apart. Press your hips forward until your torso forms a straight line from head to hips. With your hands under your shoulders, bend your elbows and lower your chest to the floor, keeping your head in line with your spine [shown]. Straighten arms to press up; repeat. Build up to 15 reps.

3

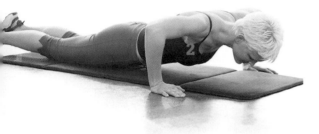

4

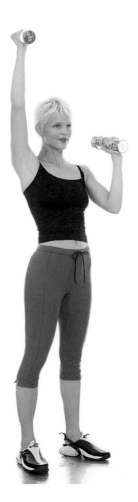

4 ALTERNATING PRESS Hold a 3- to 5-pound dumbbell in each hand and stand with your feet shoulder-width apart, abs contracted so your spine forms a straight line from head to hips. Bring the dumbbells to shoulder height, elbows bent and pointing toward the floor, palms facing in. Lift your right arm toward the ceiling without locking your elbow [shown]. Slowly lower and repeat with the opposite arm. Alternate for 10–15 reps with each arm.

The core workout
Four exercises that will recondition those muscles most taxed during pregnancy.

Now that you've gained some strength and endurance, it's time to start working your core: the abs, back, butt and hips. The following ball workout features four exercises that focus on these muscles. An added bonus: Movements done while balancing on the ball also will start to define your waist. Do 10 to 15 reps of each exercise, using a 55- to 65-centimeter stability ball, depending on your height.

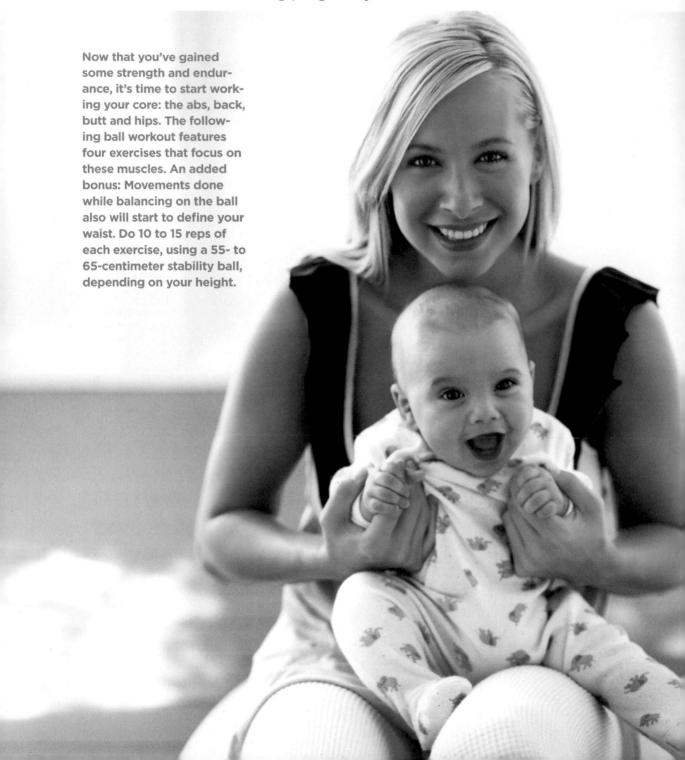

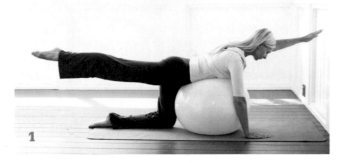

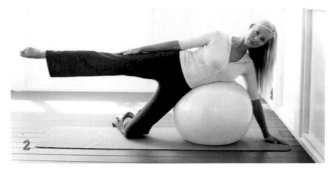

1 **SUPERWOMAN** Kneel facing the ball and drape your torso over it. Place your hands on the floor in front of the ball, your neck in line with your hips. Inhale, then exhale as you extend your left arm in front of you and your right leg behind you [shown]. Hold for 1 full breath. Inhale and lower to starting position, then exhale as you repeat with the opposite arm and leg. (This is 1 rep.)

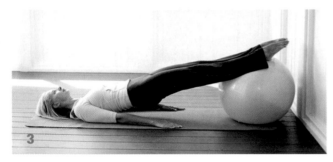

2 **SIDE LEG LIFT** Drape your left side over the ball and place your left hand on the floor. Extend your right leg straight out to the side, resting the foot lightly on the floor, right hand on thigh. Keeping your hips and shoulders steady, inhale, then exhale as you lift your right leg to hip height [shown]. Hold for 1 full breath. Slowly lower your foot to the floor; complete reps. Switch sides and repeat.

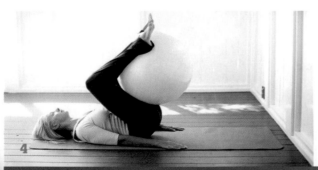

3 **BALL BRIDGE** Lie on your back and place your calves and heels on the ball, legs straight, arms at your sides, palms down. Inhale, then exhale as you squeeze your buttocks and press your lower legs and heels into the ball, lifting your hips until your body forms a straight line from shoulders to heels [shown]. Hold for 1 full breath. Slowly lower your body to starting position; complete reps.

4 **REVERSE CURL** Lie on your back, legs gripping the ball, arms extended at your sides, palms down. Draw your abs in so your lower back is in contact with the floor. Inhale, then exhale as you use your abs to lift the ball [shown]. Slowly lower the ball to the floor, keeping your abs drawn in and your lower back in contact with the floor. Complete reps.

✳ Oh, my aching back

Approximately 40 percent of women report some back pain in the weeks after delivery. Weight gain during pregnancy as well as the constant hunching over to feed, change and carry the baby around after delivery contribute to a sore back. "Simply focusing on not slouching while nursing or carrying the baby is a great way to get some relief," says Karen Nordahl, M.D., a clinical associate instructor in the department of family practice at the University of British Columbia Faculty of Medicine, who also suggests strengthening your core muscles. A heating pad can also help, as can a back massage. If the pain doesn't subside, try taking ibuprofen or acetaminophen; both are safe even if you are nursing.

Day one abdominal moves
Targeted ab exercises gentle enough
to do the day after you deliver.

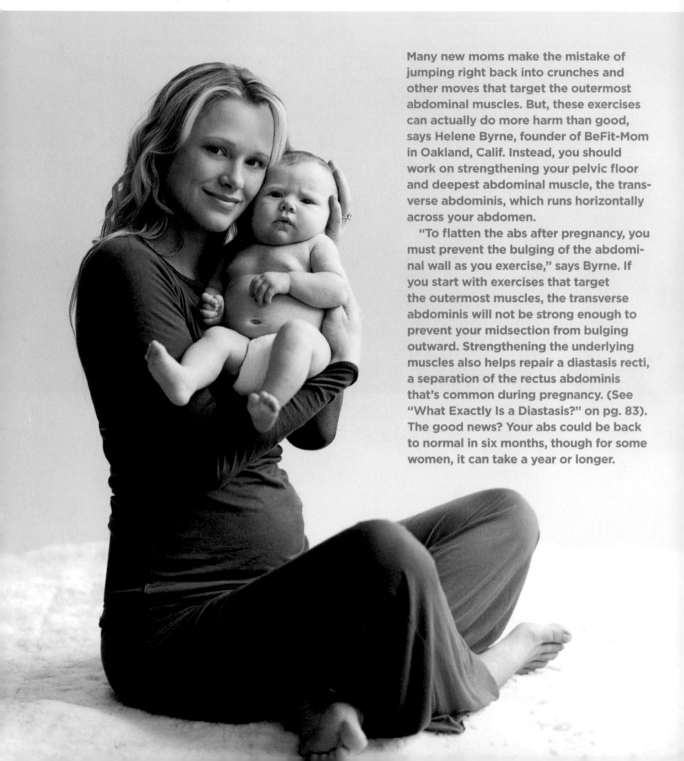

Many new moms make the mistake of
jumping right back into crunches and
other moves that target the outermost
abdominal muscles. But, these exercises
can actually do more harm than good,
says Helene Byrne, founder of BeFit-Mom
in Oakland, Calif. Instead, you should
work on strengthening your pelvic floor
and deepest abdominal muscle, the transverse abdominis, which runs horizontally
across your abdomen.

   "To flatten the abs after pregnancy, you
must prevent the bulging of the abdominal wall as you exercise," says Byrne. If
you start with exercises that target
the outermost muscles, the transverse
abdominis will not be strong enough to
prevent your midsection from bulging
outward. Strengthening the underlying
muscles also helps repair a diastasis recti,
a separation of the rectus abdominis
that's common during pregnancy. (See
"What Exactly Is a Diastasis?" on pg. 83).
The good news? Your abs could be back
to normal in six months, though for some
women, it can take a year or longer.

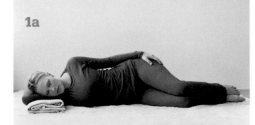

1a

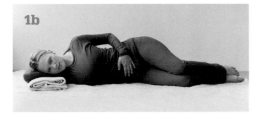

1b

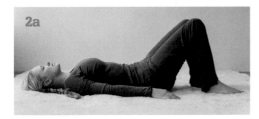

2a

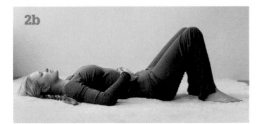

2b

The following three exercises strengthen your deepest abdominal muscle, the transverse abdominis, which (ideally) acts as an internal "girdle," giving your abs a flat appearance.

Follow this exercise program for four to six weeks. While the moves are gentle enough to do daily immediately after your baby arrives, if you had a C-section, you should wait about four to six weeks. You also should check with your doctor before beginning this or any exercise program.

1 **BELLY LACING** Lie on your right side, head resting on a folded towel, knees bent and legs together. Relax your abs completely as you inhale, then exhale through your mouth (make a hissing sound through your teeth), and slowly contract your abs while drawing your lower belly in as far as you can [A]. Place your top hand below your belly button and gently use your fingertips to draw your ab muscles in deeper [B]. Hold for a count of 3, breathing normally. Release and repeat 4 more times. Switch to the left side and repeat the sequence.

2 **BELLY SCOOPING** Lie on your back, knees bent and feet flat. Keeping your buttocks and legs relaxed, inhale, then exhale and draw your deep abdominal muscles in toward your spine, tilting your pelvis up and gently touching your lower back to the floor [A]. Place your hands on your belly, and use your fingertips to gently draw the lower ab muscles in even more while contracting them [B]. Hold for a count of 3, breathing normally, then release. Repeat 4 more times.

3 **DYNAMIC TUCK** Lie on your back, knees bent and feet flat, arms by your sides, palms down. Keeping your buttocks and legs relaxed, inhale, then exhale and draw your deep abdominal muscles in toward your spine, bringing your right knee toward your chest [A]. Using your abdominal muscles, slowly bring your left knee toward your chest, pressing your arms and hands into the floor [B]. Hold for a count of 10, then slowly release, one leg at a time, keeping abs drawn in. Repeat 4 more times, starting with your right leg.

What exactly is a diastasis?

WHAT IT IS A separation of the rectus abdominis, the "six pack" abdominal muscles, at the horizontal midline. It's caused by the force of the uterus pushing against the abdominal wall and pregnancy hormones that soften connective tissue.

HOW TO CHECK FOR IT Lie on your back with knees bent, feet flat. Place one hand behind your head and the fingertips of your other hand horizontally just below your bellybutton. Gently press your fingers into your abdominal muscles do a "crunch" by contracting your abdominal muscles and bringing your ribs toward your hips. Move your fingertips back and forth. If you feel a separation between the muscles more than two to three fingers wide or if you see a small mound protruding, you have a diastasis.

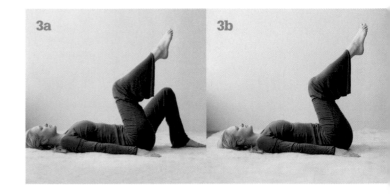

3a

3b

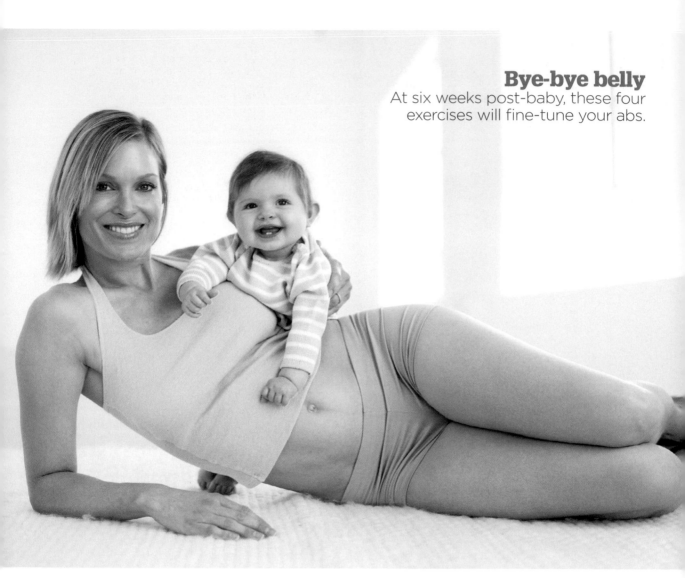

Bye-bye belly

At six weeks post-baby, these four
exercises will fine-tune your abs.

For a more challenging abdominal workout, you can begin this routine
as early as six weeks after having your baby (longer if you had a Cesarean section). If you have a diastasis, wait until the muscle separation is
less than the width of two fingers. Be sure to get your doctor's approval
before beginning this or any exercise program.

   Begin gradually: Start with eight to 10 repetitions of exercises 1 and
2, building up to 15. When you can do 15 reps of each with proper form,
add exercises 3 and 4, but reduce all reps to 10. Slowly increase your
reps; when you can complete 15 of all four exercises with proper form,
add another set of 15 reps, resting 60 seconds between sets.

1 **NO-CHEATING CHAIR ABS** Lie faceup on the floor, knees bent, lower legs resting on a chair, feet relaxed. Fold forearms behind head, hands resting on arms. Draw your abdominals up and in, then lift your head, neck and shoulders off the floor, keeping buttocks and legs relaxed [shown]. Slowly lower to starting position.

2 **SUPER-CRUNCH** Lie faceup on the floor, knees bent, feet flat on the floor. Place hands, unclasped, behind head. Draw abs up and in, and lift head, neck and shoulders off the floor. At the same time, lift knees up and bring them to meet your elbows, lifting hips slightly off the floor [shown]. Slowly lower to starting position.

3 **SUPPORTED BENT-KNEE CURL** Lie faceup on the floor, knees bent, calves parallel to the floor. Place hands behind thighs. Press legs away from you, using your hands as resistance; at the same time, draw your abs up and in, and lift your head, neck and shoulders off the floor [shown]. Slowly lower to starting position.

4 **BICYCLE** Lie faceup on the floor, knees bent, calves parallel to the floor, hands behind your head. Draw your abs up and in. Extend your left leg out; at the same time, rotate left shoulder toward right knee, lifting your head, neck and shoulders off the floor [shown]. Return to starting position and alternate with opposite leg and shoulder.

1

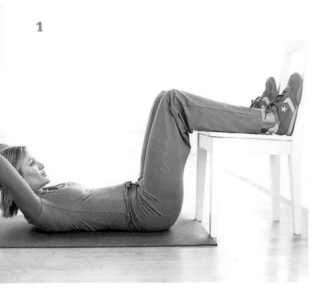

2

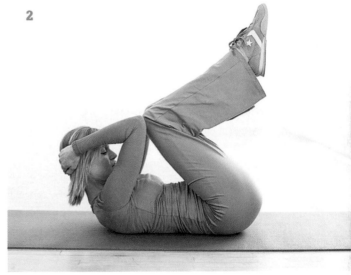

3

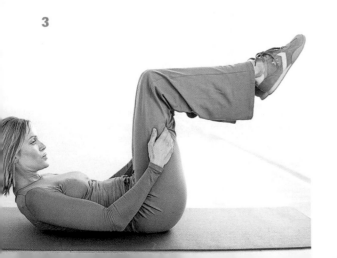

4

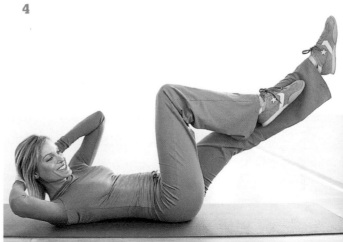

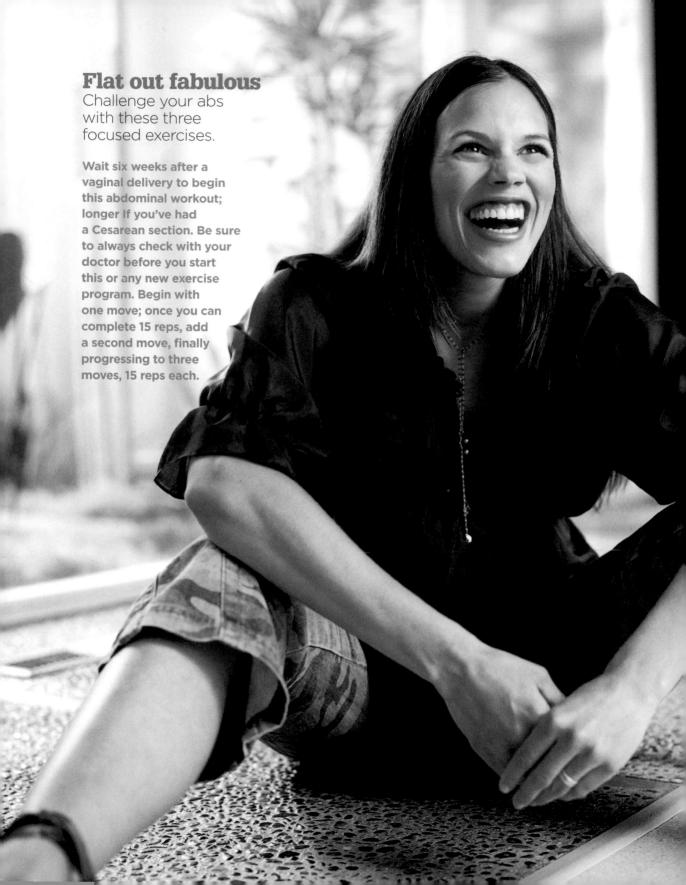

Flat out fabulous

Challenge your abs
with these three
focused exercises.

Wait six weeks after a
vaginal delivery to begin
this abdominal workout;
longer If you've had
a Cesarean section. Be sure
to always check with your
doctor before you start
this or any new exercise
program. Begin with
one move; once you can
complete 15 reps, add
a second move, finally
progressing to three
moves, 15 reps each.

1 **REVERSE CURL** Lie on your back, knees bent. With your arms at your sides, slowly lift your legs, one at a time, so that your hips and knees form 90-degree angles [A]. Gently pressing your arms into the floor, inhale, then exhale deeply as you use your abs to draw your knees into your chest. Hold, continuing to exhale [B]. Inhale and slowly return to the starting position, with hips at a 90-degree angle.

2 **SEATED BAND CURL** Place a flat band vertically on the seat and back of a chair. Grasp the top end of the band with both hands, sit on the band and line it up with your spine. Once seated, point your elbows up, keeping your feet flat on the floor. Move your hands down the band until it offers some resistance [A]. Inhale, then exhale and curl your spine, drawing your abs in and up [B]. Slowly return to an upright position.

3 **FOREARM PLANK** From a kneeling position, place your forearms on the floor with hands laced, abs drawn in [A]. Slowly lift your knees off the floor, one at a time, until your body forms a straight line from head to hips. Keep your butt tight and breathe normally [B]. Hold for 2 full breaths, then lower knees to starting position

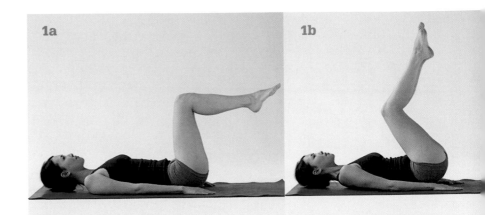

1a

1b

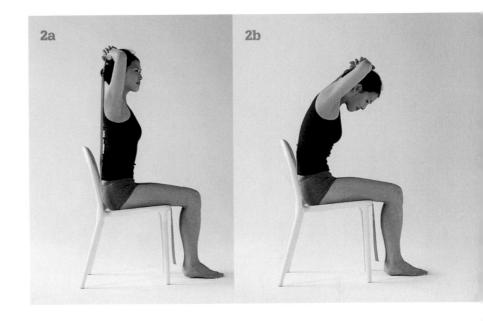

2a

2b

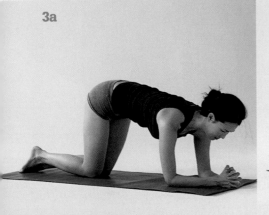

3a

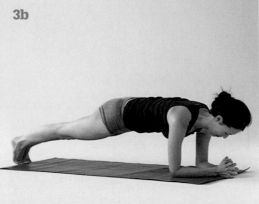

3b

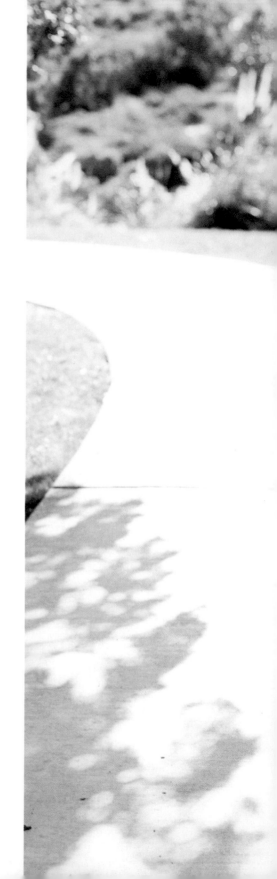

On the road again

A stroller workout is a great way to work out with your baby and bond with other moms.

What's the best way to exercise as a new mom? With your baby, of course! Pushing a stroller with the added weight of your baby (and all his gear) turns a simple walk into a fat-burning and endurance-building activity. It also gives you an opportunity to bond with your baby—and other new moms. Make a walking date with a fellow mom in your neighborhood: By getting together with other parents, you can help to combat the new-mom feelings of loneliness, isolation and exhaustion. Or sign up for a stroller-based exercise class. Designed to bring new moms together and boost your workout, classes typically include a mix of walking and strength training using water bottles or even your baby as weight. (To find a program, visit: strollerfit.com, strollerstrides.com, strollercize.com or babybootcamp.com.)

The following Strollercize workout, designed by Naples, Fla.-based trainer Elizabeth Trindade will strengthen your whole body. You can start it at six weeks postpartum, or earlier with your doctor's approval. Do 20 minutes of striding with your baby in the stroller, then perform the four moves on pgs. 90–93. Try to get in two or more sessions per week, taking at least one day off in between.

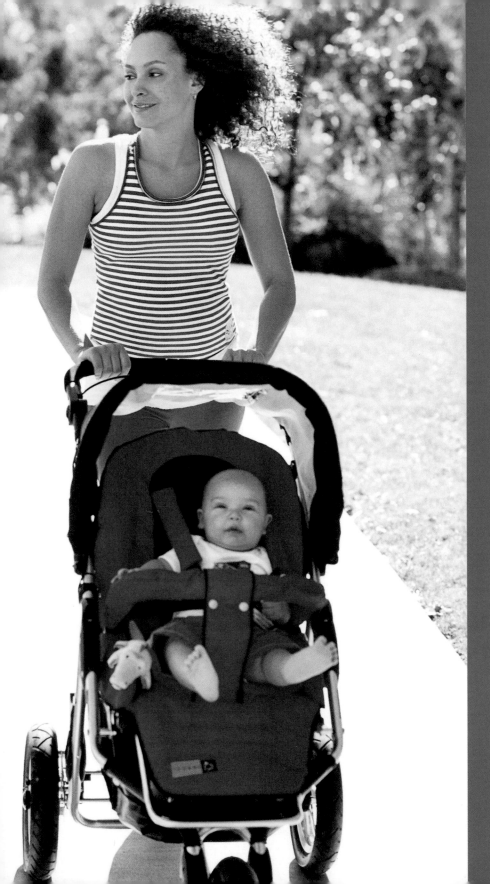

Get by with a little help from your mom friends

Women who gather at the neighborhood tot lot may be practicing an important evolutionary behavior. Animal research suggests that mothers who spend time with female friends increase their babies' chances of long-term survival.

The study was based on 16 years of observations of baboon tribes in Kenya, where researchers found that the more time female baboons spent with other females—particularly while grooming themselves and each other—the more likely their offspring were to survive until their first birthdays.

Scientists aren't sure why such social bonds affect infant survival. It could be because large groups of baboons can better ward off predators or because social isolation contributes to illness. For human moms, pushing strollers alongside other moms or meeting for coffee at the local cafe may serve the same purpose.

Warm up

Begin with three minutes of gentle exercises, such as ankle rolls, side-to-side lunges and shoulder circles, to limber up your joints and muscles. Follow the warm-up session with a 20-minute walk with your baby in a stroller. Vary your pace and intensity throughout the walk for the most effective work-out. A good indicator of how hard to push yourself is the talk test: Walk at a pace that keeps your heart rate up, but allows you to carry on a conversation.

Build strength

At six to 12 weeks post-partum, do 10 reps of each of the exercises shown here after your 20-minute stroller walk. Three to four months after delivering, do 15 reps; after four or more months postpartum, do 20 reps and add a set of 5 push-ups and 5 planks, holding the plank position for 10 to 20 seconds.

Cool down

Sit on a bench and stretch all your muscles, especially your hamstrings, calves and lower back. Hold each stretch for 10 to 15 seconds.

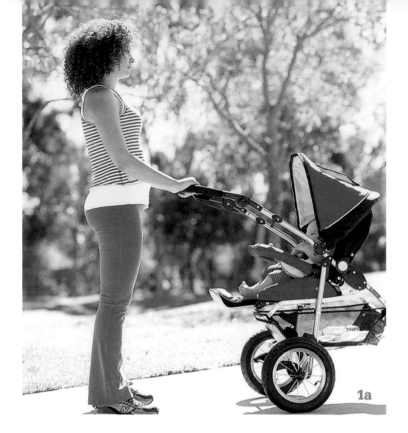

1a

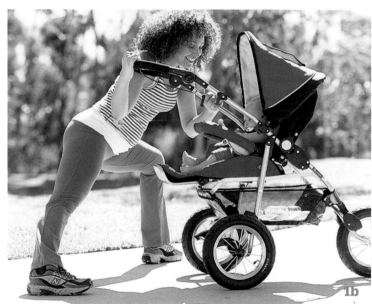

1b

1 PEEKABOO With your feet hip-width apart, face the stroller, holding the handle with both hands [A]. Take a wide step forward and to the left with your left leg, bending your knee to lean beyond the side of the stroller; keep your right leg straight. Staying low, peek around the stroller at your baby [B], then shift your body weight back, straightening your left knee to return to the starting position. Alternate sides, and complete reps.

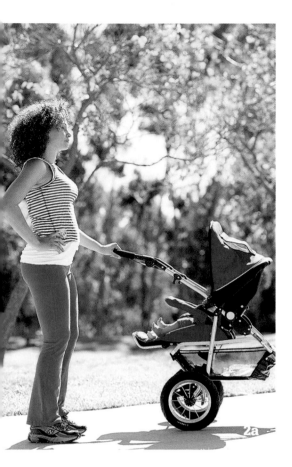

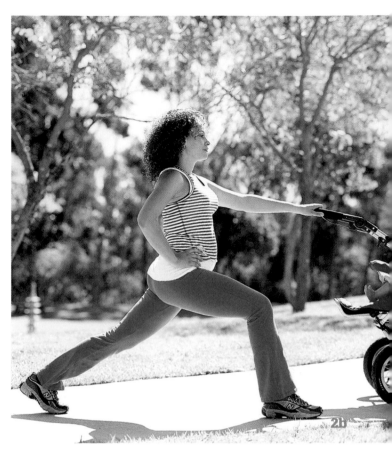

2 **STROLLER-LUNGE WALKS** Stand behind and slightly to the right of the stroller. Place your left hand on the center of the handle, right hand on your hip. Contract your abdominal muscles so that your tailbone points down **[A]**. Take a long step forward with your right foot, bending your knee until it is almost over the ankle; keep your left leg fairly straight. At the same time, push the stroller forward **[B]**. Next, push off the back foot so your feet are together again. Complete reps with right leg, then switch and do reps with left leg, holding the handle with your right hand.

Put safety first

You can take an easy walk with your friends before your six-week postpartum checkup, but wait for your doctor's approval before beginning this or any other postnatal strength program.

BE PREPARED Make sure your baby is fed and bring sunscreen for yourself and your baby. Most experts recommend protecting your baby with a hat, clothing and shade, too.

USE GOOD FORM When holding the stroller handles, keep your wrists straight, elbows bent slightly outward. Don't grip too tightly. Take long strides and stand tall with your abdominals drawn in, shoulders back and down and chest lifted. When walking forward, strike the ground with your heel and roll through your foot and be sure to watch for obstacles ahead of you.

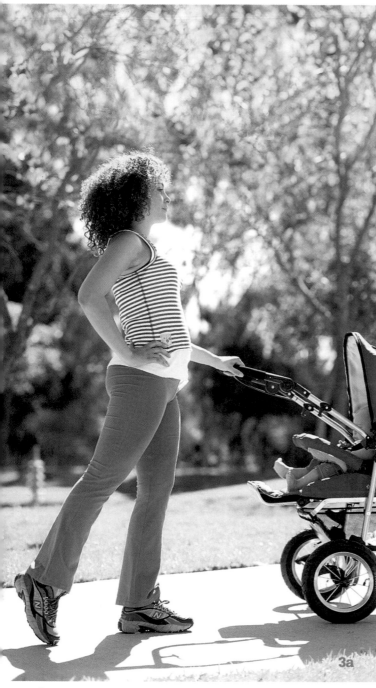
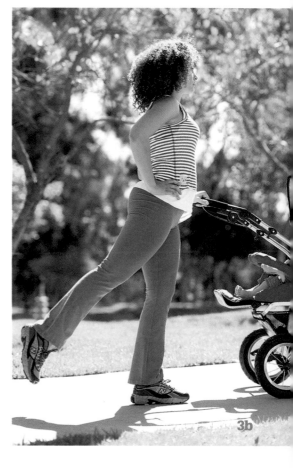

3a

3b

3 **ARABESQUE BUTTOCKS PULSE** Grasping the handle with your left hand, stand behind and slightly to the right of the stroller. Stand on your left foot, leg straight, and extend your right leg behind you, toes touching the ground [A]. Lift your right leg about 4 inches and pulse it upward for the desired number of reps [B]. Switch sides and repeat with your left leg.

Mood boost: a walk in the park

New mothers suffering from the "baby blues" may find relief by stroller-walking with their babies. This is due in part to the fact that exercise itself acts as an antidepressant, as researchers discovered when studying participants in stroller-walking classes. If the activity is vigorous enough, it might help by stimulating the brain's production of endorphins, biochemicals that can inspire a sense of well-being. Or depressed moms may simply find that regular exercise increases their self-esteem and that the ensuing weight loss and improved muscle tone also lift their spirits. If nothing else, new mothers benefit from the break time or distraction from stress a brisk stroll provides.

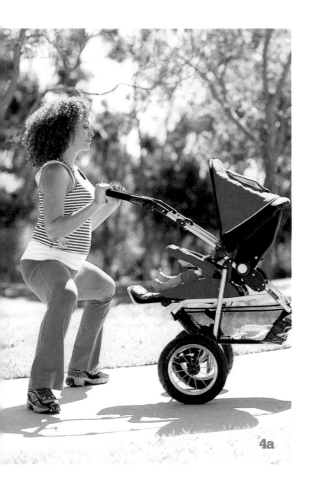

4a

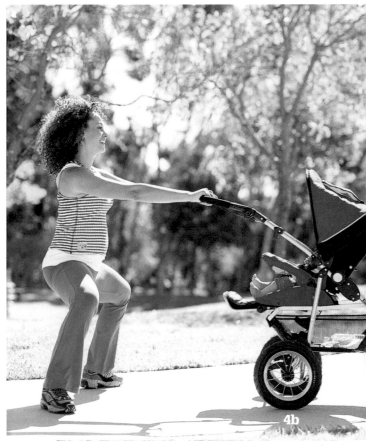

4b

4 **MOMENT OF PEACE** Face the stroller and place your hands far apart on the handle, toes facing out. Move into a wide plié: Contract your abs, bend your knees and lower your torso, keeping your heels on the ground; you'll feel a stretch on the inside of your thighs [A]. Push the stroller away from you and hold it at arm's length for a count of 20 [B]. Slowly roll the stroller back toward you. Straighten your body and repeat.

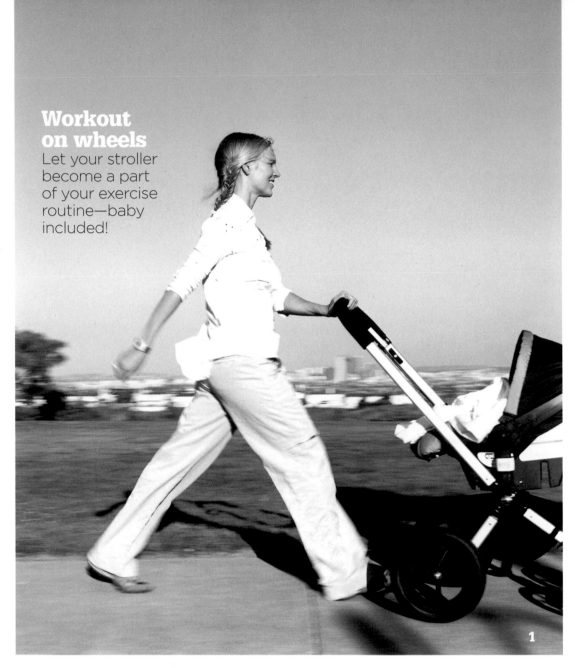

Workout on wheels

Let your stroller become a part of your exercise routine—baby included!

The six moves featured here add up to an easy and fun 30-minute circuit-style stroller workout that combines five-minute cardiovascular intervals with one- to two-minute toning sessions. Before you begin, you will need three full 16.9-ounces or larger water bottles—one for drinking and two to use as weights. Wait six weeks after a vaginal delivery to begin this workout; longer if you've had a Cesarean section. Always check with your doctor before starting this or any workout program.

1 MOM ON A MISSION
[Cardio: 5 minutes] As you walk, extend each leg as far forward as possible, without sacrificing form. Occasionally, try pushing the stroller with one hand and move the other arm alongside your body in the opposite direction as your forward leg without swinging it out of control [Shown].

Stroller power

Walking with a stroller can increase the intensity of your exercise routine by 15 to 20 percent, according to a study from the University of Wisconsin-La Crosse. "Women can get a good workout pushing a stroller," says John Porcari, Ph.D., co-author of the study and a professor in the department of exercise and sports science. Researchers found that 30 minutes of walking at a moderate pace (3.5 mph) with a stroller burned 222 calories, the equivalent of 30 minutes of cycling at 10 mph or playing tennis.

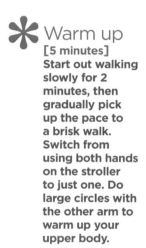

✳ Warm up
[5 minutes]
Start out walking slowly for 2 minutes, then gradually pick up the pace to a brisk walk. Switch from using both hands on the stroller to just one. Do large circles with the other arm to warm up your upper body.

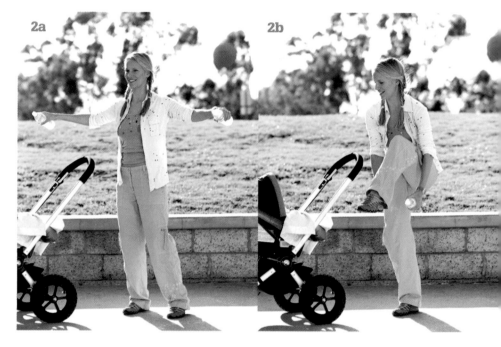
2a   2b

2 PATTY CAKE **[Toning: 1–2 minutes]** Lock the stroller and grab two full water bottles. Stand facing your baby with feet hip-width apart, knees slightly bent and arms extended at shoulder-height, palms down **[A]**. Exhale and raise your left knee to your chest, touching the bottles together under your knee **[B]**. Switch legs and repeat for a total of 10 repetitions, working up to 20. Count out loud or talk to your baby as you do the move.

3 STROLL 'N' SKIP **[Cardio: 5 minutes]** Walk briskly for 1 minute. Then, holding the stroller with your right hand, move toward the left side of the stroller taking large skips. Bring your knee up toward your chest as you swing your left arm up and out, in opposition to your knee. Switch sides and continue to skip, alternating sides. Walk in the middle, as needed, to catch your breath **[not shown]**.

EXERCISE AFTER BABY

95

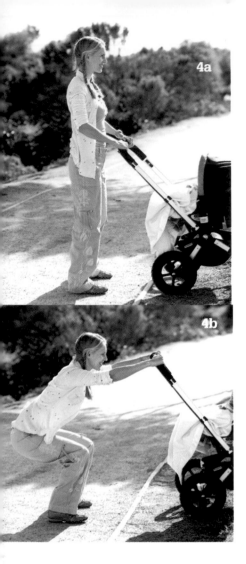

4a

4b

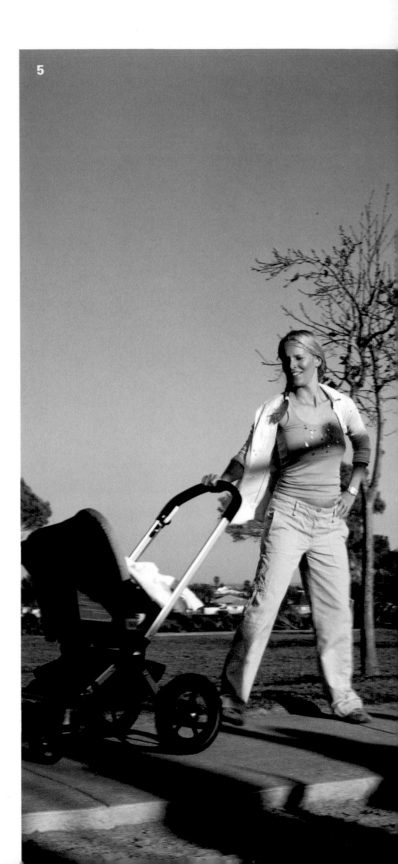

5

4 SIT 'N' ROLL [Toning: 1–2 minutes] Stand with your feet hip-width apart and toes pointing straight ahead. Hold onto the stroller for balance, elbows bent, abs drawn in, shoulders back and down [A]. Keeping weight on your heels, bend your knees into a squat until your thighs are as parallel to the ground as possible, leaning your torso forward at a 45-degree angle. Keep your knees over ankles and straighten your arms, letting the stroller roll away from you [B]. Straighten your legs and return to the starting position, bringing the stroller back toward you. Do 10 reps, building up to 20.

5 GALLOPING GAL **[Cardio: 5 minutes]** Walk straight for 1 minute. Then, turn your right side to the stroller, your right hand holding the handle, left hand on hip. Take big steps sideways, looking over your right shoulder **[shown]**. Place your feet farther than hip-width apart and bend knees into a semi-squat. Straighten legs and "gallop" to the right, moving your feet together and apart in a quick cadence for 30 seconds. Repeat gallop for 30 seconds on the left side. Alternate 1 minute of walking straight ahead with 1 minute of galloping.

6 ROCK-A-BYE **[Toning: 1–2 minutes]** Stand with the locked stroller to your right and turned sideways. Hold a full water bottle in your left hand, elbow bent, right hand holding the handle, feet hip-width apart and abs drawn in **[A]**. Bend your left knee and step back into a lunge with the right foot, leaning your torso forward and straightening your left arm behind you **[B]**. Return to starting position and complete 10 reps, working up to 20, then switch sides.

Cool down [1–2 minutes]

Walk slowly for 2 minutes, then stretch your calves, quads, hamstrings, lower back and shoulders, holding each stretch for approximately 30 seconds without bouncing.

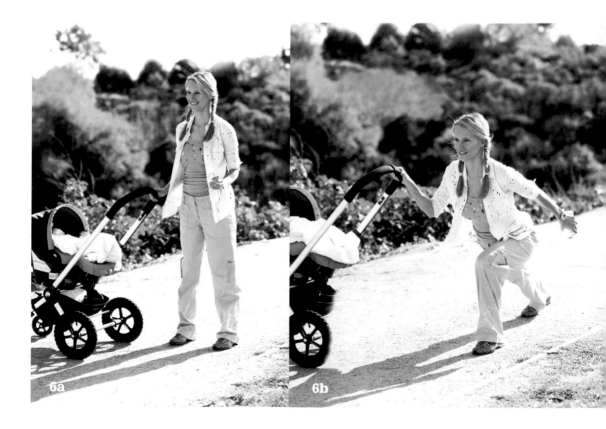

6a   6b

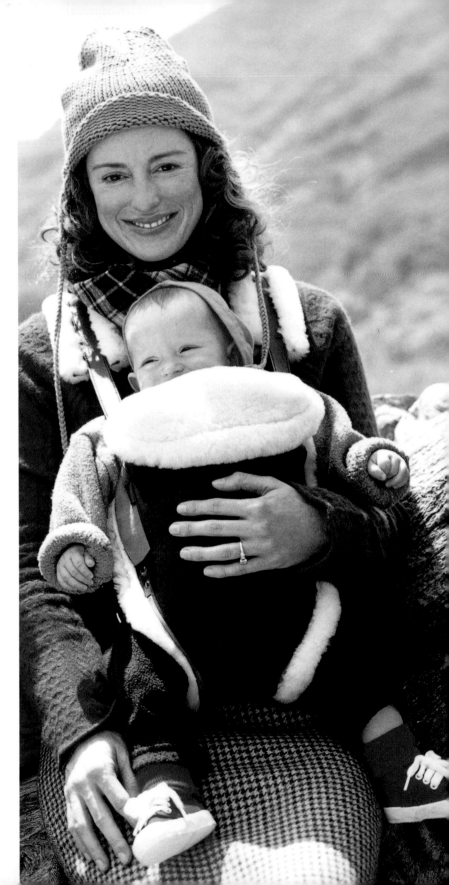

Take a hike

What's the best place to work off the baby weight? The great outdoors.

Hiking not only helps build strength, but it also allows you to get out with your baby and other new parents. Start by finding a few hiking partners. Check out new mom groups, gyms, churches, childbirth-education classes or local outdoor-gear stores.

The following workout is challenging; if you didn't keep up a regular exercise routine during pregnancy, reduce the hiking times to those that feel most comfortable for you.

DAYS 1-14 With your doctor's approval, begin by walking about two blocks to a quarter-mile twice a week, depending on your strength, with your baby in a front carrier. Stay on flat ground as you regain strength and balance, and wear well-cushioned shoes and thick cotton socks. (If you've had a Cesarean section and find wearing a front carrier uncomfortable, use a stroller.)

DAYS 15-28 After two weeks on flat terrain, add short staircases or small hills (they will help build your butt and calf muscles). Increase the distance as you get stronger. To build strength, increase hiking to four times a week, 30 minutes per hike.

AFTER 4 WEEKS You now may be ready to undertake a more rigorous hiking routine (check with your doctor first, of course). Be sure to stretch all major muscle groups before and after each hike.

4–6 WEEKS During these two weeks, build up to an hour-long hike. To build strength and stamina, alternate hilly terrain with flat: On Monday, Wednesday and Friday, hike on trails with small hills. On Tuesday and Thursday, keep to flat ground.

6–8 WEEKS For the next two weeks, extend your hiking time by 15–20 minutes per hike, and drop a day so that you're hiking four times a week.

8–12 WEEKS For these four weeks, extend your hiking time another 30–45 minutes and drop a day, so you're hiking for two hours, three days per week, still varying days on flat ground with days hiking on hills. On the two days that you're not hiking, do a different exercise, such as aerobics or swimming, to stay active. (When your baby weighs 16 pounds, it may be time to transfer her from a front carrier to a backpack.)

Do it right

WALK NATURALLY Push forward with your hips and pull in your abdominal muscles. Doing this will help to keep yourself balanced and your back supported.

STAND TALL It's easy to lean forward while wearing a backpack. Avoid this by keeping your hips forward and your shoulders relaxed.

USE PROPER FORM ON HILLS When walking downhill, keep your knees slightly bent and take small steps, rolling from heel to toe. When walking uphill or downhill while wearing a front carrier, shorten your stride and swing your arms as you would normally without a carrier.

MOVE YOUR ARMS Raise your arms over your head from time to time. Doing this will keep your hands and fingers from swelling.

USE THE BUDDY SYSTEM Never hike alone and bring your cellphone for emergencies.

KEEP IT UP! Even if you return to work after your maternity leave, try to keep hiking, at least as a weekend family activity.

Protect your baby

AVOID THE HEAT Don't take your baby hiking on very hot days; overheating can be dangerous for both you and your baby.

KEEP 'EM COVERED When hiking together, make sure your baby is completely protected from the sun's rays. Dress her in lightweight clothes that cover her arms and legs, and use a sun hat, umbrella or canopy as well. Liberal amounts of children's sunscreen are OK for babies older than 6 months; for younger babies, apply sparingly to exposed areas, such as her face and hands.

PREPARE FOR WET WEATHER A little rain never hurt anyone. If you get stuck in a shower, zip your rain jacket around your baby or use an umbrella.

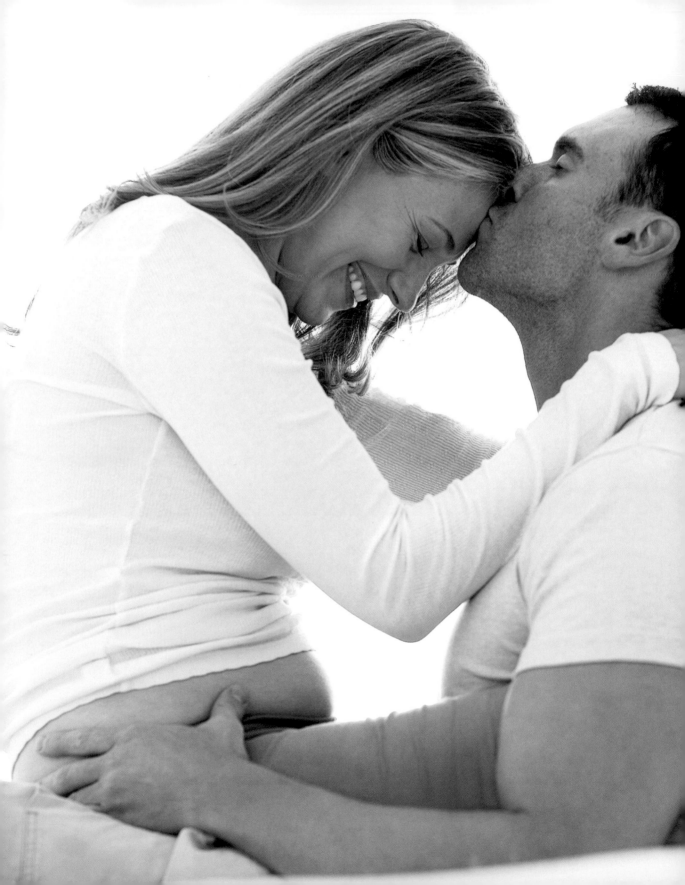

With a newborn in the house, sex is likely the last thing on your priority list. And, for many couples, the added responsibility of caring for a baby is often the root of new conflicts in your relationship. The good news? It happens to almost every set of new parents and it's only temporary—if you take the necessary steps to rekindle your love life and work out your differences.

The following chapter offers tips to making sex fun again, as well as a postpartum workout that will shape up your pelvic floor—and rev up your love life! Plus, you'll get a dad's point of view on life after baby, as well as learn the best ways to resolve disagreements and reconnect with your partner.

L ost that lovin' feeling? Since the birth of your baby, you may have found that your libido has gone missing and wonder if it will ever reappear. And while your sexual derailment may be baffling, rest assured that what you're experiencing is normal, and that with time, you and your partner will find your way back to each other. Here, the reasons behind your dry spell, plus tips for getting back into the groove.

Why you don't want it

Most women tend to lose interest in sex following childbirth—and, potentially, throughout their baby's first year, says OB-GYN Gregory R. Moore, M.D., M.P.H., adjunct associate professor of obstetrics and gynecology at the University of Kentucky Medical School in Lexington. And it's no wonder: You're coping with physical recovery from both the pregnancy and birth, the 24/7 demands of new motherhood, sleep deprivation, body-image issues and hormonal shifts that result from childbirth and breastfeeding. "Plus," Moore adds, "there's a third person in the room—a baby."

Even after your doctor gives you the go-ahead to resume your sex life—usually at six weeks postpartum, longer if you had a Cesarean section (see "When Is It Safe to Have Sex Again?" pg. 103)—you still may not be raring to go, especially if you're nursing. "The decrease in libido is partially hormonal because estrogen levels drop radically after childbirth and stay low during breastfeeding," says Suzanne Merrill-Nach, M.D., an OB-GYN in San Diego. "Drops in estrogen cause a thinning of the vaginal wall and a decrease in vaginal secretions, and since estrogen is one of the hormones involved in a woman's sexuality, that makes for a definite libido stopper."

Maternal anxiety is another big mood dampener. Your senses have been reorganized to be highly attuned to the baby: Was that a cry? How can I be sure he's breathing? Is he positioned safely in the crib? Won't he need to nurse soon? So even when you feel rested and make an attempt at intimacy, your biology can conspire against you. The complexities of breastfeeding and dealing with a new, post-baby body are at play in a new mother's sexual identity. You might have extra pregnancy weight, residual discomfort

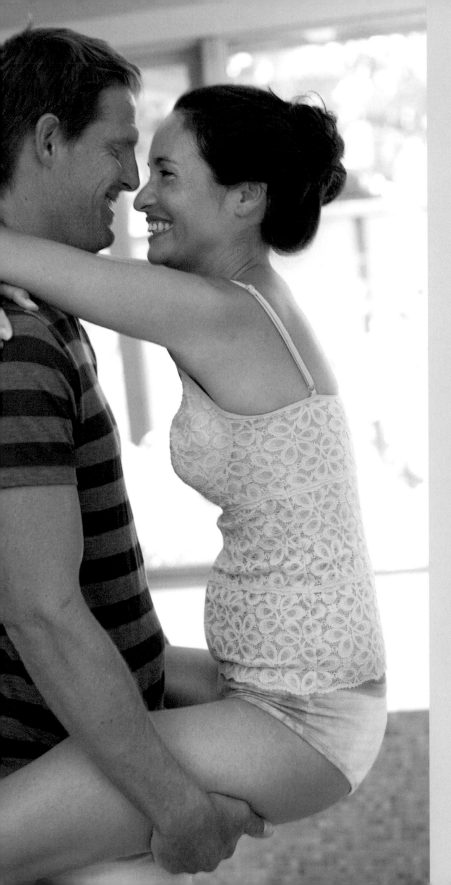

When is it safe to have sex again?

Most OBs recommend that women postpone sex for at least six weeks after giving birth, even longer after a Cesarean section. Women who delivered vaginally are at risk for infection as the cervix closes, the uterus contracts and the uterine lining and vaginal tissues heal. And if you underwent a C-section, you need even more time to avoid stressing the internal sutures holding your abdominal muscles together (external stitches will have been removed within about a week of delivery). You also don't want to add pressure and discomfort to healing scar tissue. "You should be able to push on the scar area and have no pain before resuming sex," says San Diego OB-GYN Suzanne Merrill-Nach, M.D.

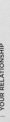

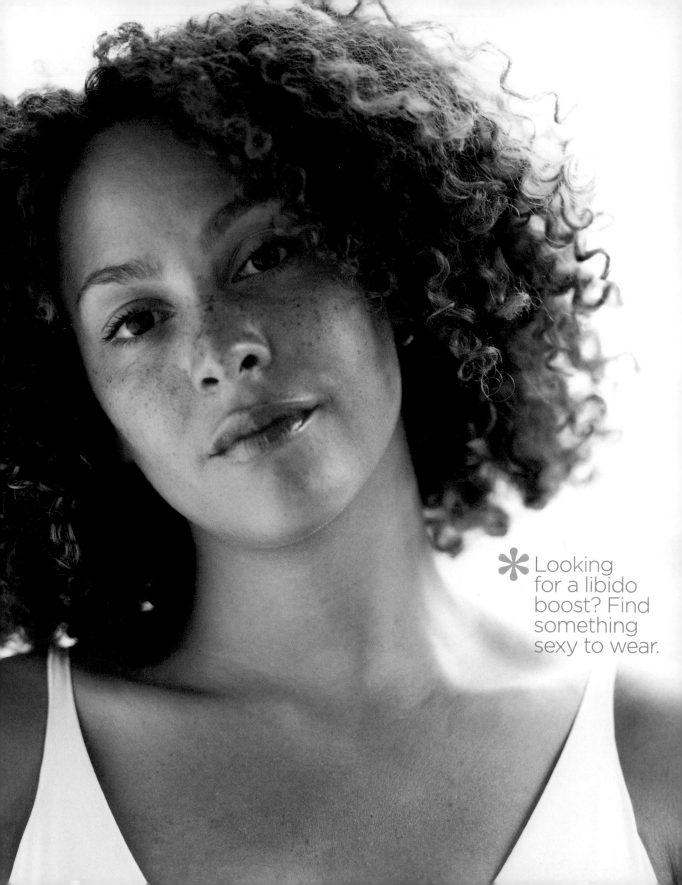

* Looking for a libido boost? Find something sexy to wear.

from delivery and leaking breasts, all of which can result in less-than-sexy sensations. Then there are the unrelenting and exhausting demands of taking care of a baby—these can make the prospect of giving physical attention to your partner seem like a chore. "Many new mothers say they feel they have two people to take care of," says Belisa Vranich, Psy.D., a clinical psychologist in New York City. "They say that both their husband and the baby want them in a physical way and that they feel groped at. Also, women need to feel sexy to have sex. But after having a baby, most women feel almost the polar opposite of sexy."

What you can do about it

Start by being patient with yourself and your partner and communicating with each other. Go ahead, Vranich says, and verbalize what you're both thinking: "Are we ever going to have sex again?" This should make you both laugh (or cry) and relieve the stress a bit. Talk about how you're feeling as you make the tremendous adjustment to motherhood, and encourage him to share his feelings about becoming a father. Some other tips:

FIND A CHILD CARE PERSON YOU TRUST so you can schedule weekly re-acquaintance time without the baby. Even though you may not be able to get away every week, try to make one-on-one time a priority, even if it's only a half-hour for a walk together.

ATTEMPT TO RECOUP LOST SLEEP by napping whenever the baby does (laundry, e-mail and dirty dishes be damned) or going to bed early—because in the sex vs. sleep battle, sleep inevitably wins.

IF YOU'RE BREASTFEEDING and ready to have sex again, consider pumping or nursing beforehand so your milk doesn't let down in the midst of the action. Breast milk is essential for your newborn, not foreplay.

TO HELP GET YOUR HEAD OUT OF "BABY SPACE," find something sexy to wear. "Even if it's a gimmick, do it—whatever it takes to make you feel sexy," Vranich says.

AS SOON AS YOU THINK YOU'RE READY, schedule some time away with your partner. "If you can get away for a weekend, do it," advises Vranich. "But agree to just sleep the first night. The next night, have sex."

Don't forget the birth control

Some experts speculate that a flagging libido following childbirth is nature's way of protecting you from getting pregnant too soon. But, when you start having intercourse, you need to use birth control. While many women think it's unlikely they'll resume ovulating and be able to conceive shortly after giving birth, this is only the case for a few months post-delivery and only if a woman is breastfeeding full time— at least every four hours around the clock. Even then, nursing is not a foolproof method of birth control. Because getting pregnant is always a possibility, many experts recommend using contraception even if you are breastfeeding; talk to your doctor about the method that is best for you.

Giving birth won't spoil your sex life

Some women worry that having a vaginal delivery might wreak havoc on their long-term ability to enjoy sex. However, a study has found that the method of delivery—vaginal, Cesarean or vaginal with forceps or vacuum—appears to have little impact on sexual activity one year after childbirth. But, a woman's sex life before delivery predicted what it would be like afterward. Dutch researchers surveyed 377 women about their sex lives at 12 weeks into the pregnancy and at one year postpartum and found that those who were not having sex early in the pregnancy were 11 times more likely to be sexually inactive one year after childbirth.

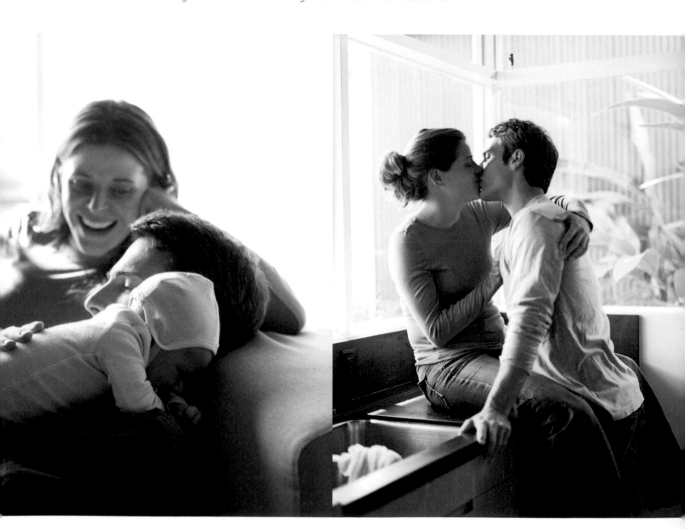

Sex after baby: your body

For many new moms, getting back to sex after having a baby is a cause for anxiety. To put your mind at ease, here's the scoop on women's biggest sex-related worries:

WORRY NO. 1: SEX WILL BE PAINFUL

REAL DEAL Having a baby causes the ligaments that support the uterus to stretch, making it slightly lower, says Mark Chag, M.D., an OB-GYN at Harbour Women's Health in Portsmouth, N.H. While discomfort caused by the penis hitting the uterus during intercourse is normal (and easily remedied by switching positions), pain is not. As long as you wait until you're given the green light by your doctor (usually six weeks), sex should be painless, Chag says. If it isn't, talk with your doctor, especially if you had an episiotomy; you could have another tear or an infection.

WORRY NO. 2: MY VAGINA WILL BE STRETCHED OUT

REAL DEAL Although the vagina obviously expands during childbirth, "it is very elastic and returns to its normal contour afterward," says urologist Jennifer Berman, M.D., director of the Berman Women's Wellness center in Los Angeles. If you're concerned about tightness, do Kegel exercises or other pelvic-muscle-strengthening moves (For a post-baby pelvic-floor workout, see pgs. 108-109). Note: Doing Kegels during intercourse can help keep your partner happy.

WORRY NO. 3: NURSING WILL MAKE MY VAGINA DRY

REAL DEAL "Because of low estrogen levels, lack of vaginal lubrication is common after delivery, especially for nursing mothers," Chag says. However, he adds, most women find the problem corrects itself once they stop breastfeeding. In the meantime, use a vaginal lubricant like K-Y Jelly. If dryness persists for longer than two months after you give birth or stop breastfeeding, talk with your OB-GYN.

WORRY NO. 4: I'LL LOOK FUNNY "DOWN THERE"

REAL DEAL While your vaginal area may be swollen after you give birth, it returns to its normal appearance within four to six weeks. "The vagina is like a rubber band," Berman says. "It'll bounce back." And so, probably, will your love life.

* After delivery, be sure to ease back into intercourse. Start with playful hugging and kissing and go from there.

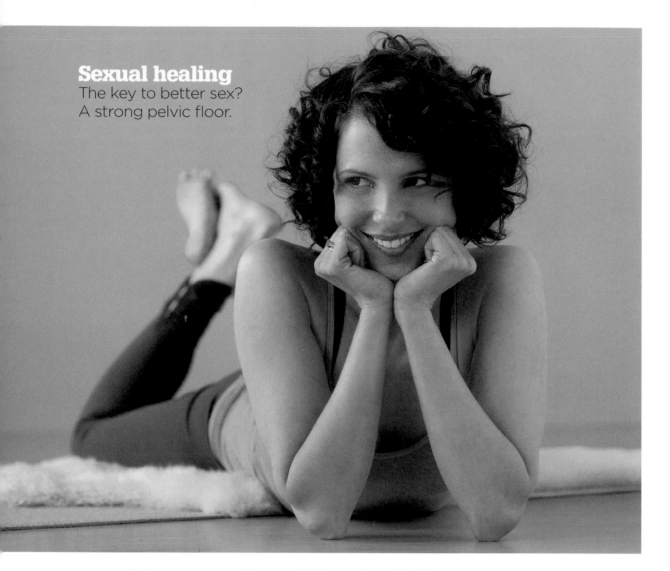

Sexual healing
The key to better sex?
A strong pelvic floor.

During pregnancy, labor and delivery, the pelvic-floor muscles are stressed and stretched, resulting in a weak pelvic floor. Just like a flabby leg or arm muscle, the pelvic floor needs exercise to regain its shape and strength, says Tasha Mulligan, a physical therapist in Urbandale, Iowa, and the creator of the DVD *Hab it: Pelvic Floor*. There's an added benefit: "The stronger your pelvic-floor muscles are, the more blood flow you have to the area," says Mulligan. "With increased blood flow, you have heightened sensitivity. And, with stronger muscles, you have more intense contractions during orgasm."

Kegel exercises are the best way to shape up your pelvic floor, but it's also important to strengthen the surrounding muscles, too, including the abdominals, hips and lower back. (To learn how to do a Kegel, see "Do Your Kegels," pg. 27.) The following workout, designed by Mulligan, can be done every other day, but wait six weeks after delivery before starting; longer if you've had a Cesarean section. Always check with your doctor before beginning this or any exercise program.

After a C-section

Even if you had a Cesarean section, your pelvic-floor muscles are likely weakened. Not only are they stressed during pregnancy, a C-section incision directly affects the abdominal muscles adjacent to the pelvic floor. Your pelvic floor can't fully function without the help of your abdominal muscles, says physical therapist Tasha Mulligan, so it's important to strengthen them both after a C-section.

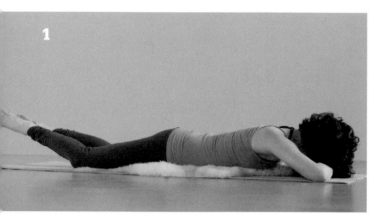

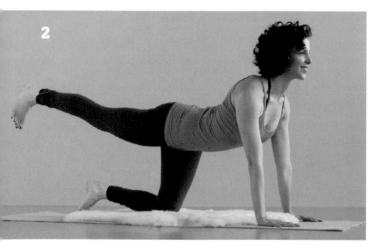

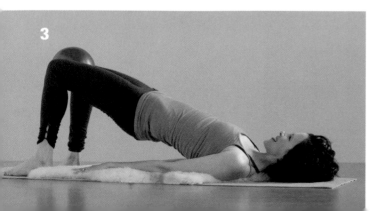

1 HEEL SQUEEZE Lie facedown, resting your forehead on your hands, knees shoulder-width apart. Bend your knees so that your feet are approximately 12 inches from the ground. Turn your toes out and bring your heels together. In this position, squeeze your buttocks as you press your heels together and do a Kegel [shown]. Hold for 2 counts, breathing normally, then release. Do 10 times, working up to 3 sets of 10.

2 LEG EXTENSIONS Get down on your hands and knees, wrists directly under your shoulders. Draw your abdominals up and in. Inhale, then exhale as you extend your right leg straight back [shown]. Hold for 2 counts as you do a Kegel. Keep your body still as you bring your right leg back to the starting position. Switch sides and repeat. Do 10 times on each side, working up to 3 sets of 10.

3 BRIDGE SQUEEZE Lie on your back with your knees bent and feet flat, arms at your sides. Place a soft, squishy ball or pillow between your knees and draw your abdominals in. Inhale, then exhale as you tighten your buttocks and lift your hips until your upper torso forms a straight line [shown]. In this position, squeeze the ball for 2 counts as you do a Kegel, then lower hips. Do 10 times, working up to 3 sets of 10.

What is the pelvic floor?

The pelvic floor is composed of four muscle layers: the anal sphincter, the urogenital triangle, the urovaginal sphincter and the levator ani. Shaped like a hammock, it links front to back, from your pubic bone to your tailbone.

When two become three

The usual advice people hear for keeping their relationship healthy hardly applies to couples who have a newborn in the house: You don't need someone telling you to enjoy regular "date nights" with your partner when you barely have the energy to change your bra, let alone sit through dinner and a movie. But even if you're low on sleep, sex, money and patience, you both have to keep going. Here are five situations that commonly test new parents—and expert advice on minimizing conflict.

1. You're always bickering about chores

WHAT'S BEHIND IT You feel as if your workload around the house has ballooned since the baby was born while his has stayed the same (and he hasn't offered to help).

RELATIONSHIP SAVER Each person should assume certain jobs so there is less chance for arguments, says marriage therapist and psychologist Terri L. Orbuch, Ph.D., a research professor at the Institute for Social Research at the University of Michigan in Ann Arbor. Divide tasks according to what each of you likes to do best. Maybe you enjoy cooking and your husband finds wielding the vacuum cleaner relaxing. Or take turns so neither of you feels stuck always doing the same thing. For example, you can vacuum the living room while your partner chops vegetables in the kitchen.

Another way to keep housework—as well as arguments—from assuming monstrous proportions is to do chores in spurts. Put your baby in an infant carrier and spend five to 15 minutes vacuuming a room, doing a load of laundry or emptying the dishwasher. Do this a few times a day—you'll be amazed at what gets done.

2. Neither of you wants the night shift

WHAT'S BEHIND IT Your partner says he needs his sleep so he can be well rested for work. You argue that you can't function and take care of the baby all day if you've been up half the night tending to an infant.

RELATIONSHIP SAVER Ask your partner to get up with the baby on weekends or when he's not facing a stressful day at work. Or sleep in shifts. For example, you can each get 7 hours of rest if you sleep from 8 p.m. to 3 a.m., and your

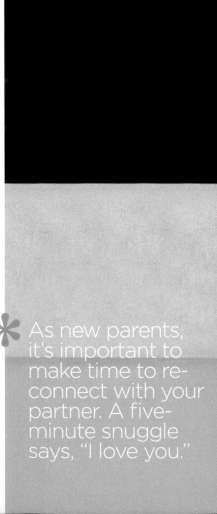

As new parents, it's important to make time to reconnect with your partner. A five-minute snuggle says, "I love you."

Bridging the distance

The hard work of raising a newborn, combined with sleep deprivation and the sudden loss of a spontaneous lifestyle, often leads to hostility between partners, according to Alyson Shapiro, Ph.D., assistant professor at the School of Social and Family Dynamics at Arizona State University in Tempe. Her advice:

STAY POSITIVE Notice what your partner is doing right and express appreciation. Also make it a priority to talk or do activities together while the baby sleeps.

HEED THE WARNING SIGNS Certain behaviors amp up marital strife; these include criticism, contempt, defensiveness and withdrawal. "Discuss problems with the intent to solve them, not to make your spouse feel bad," says Shapiro.

GET SOME SHUT-EYE You're never at your best when sleep-deprived. You and your partner should aim to get at least two three-hour periods of rest every 24 hours as soon as possible after the baby is born.

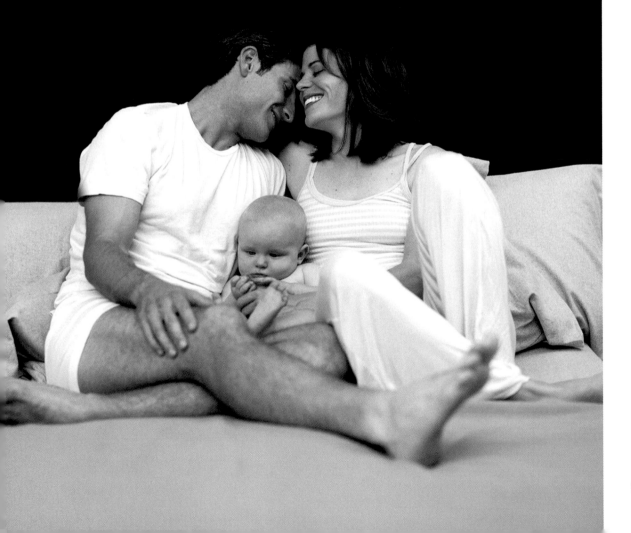

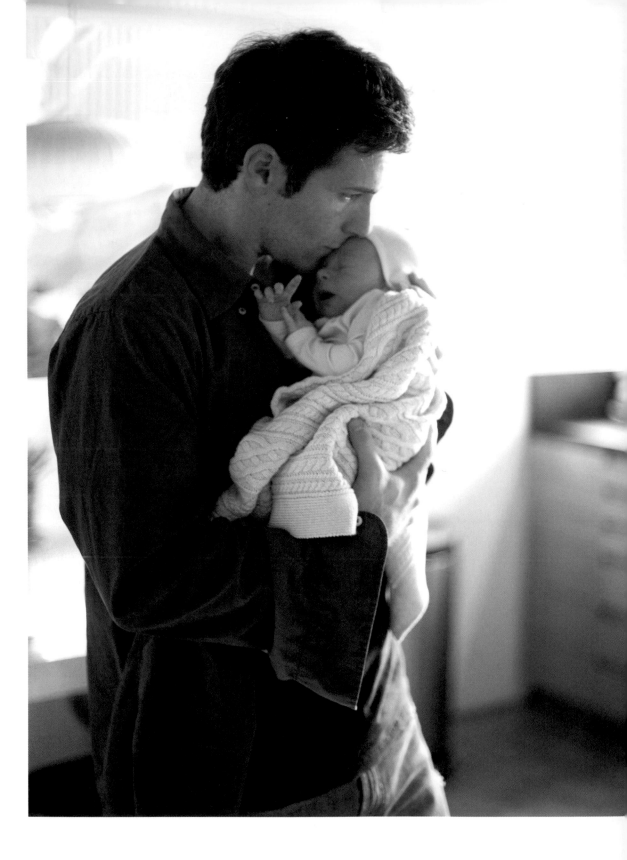

partner snoozes from midnight to 7 a.m. If you are nursing, pump before going to bed so your partner can give the baby a bottle of breast milk during his shift.

3. You're constantly criticizing his baby-care techniques

WHAT'S BEHIND IT Nervousness and insecurity about having responsibility for a newborn; the need to control what's largely uncontrollable (an infant).

RELATIONSHIP SAVER If you snap at him every time you think he's not holding the bottle at the precise correct angle or swaddling the baby exactly right, take a deep breath and realize that there is no one correct way to do things. As long as your baby is safe, don't create conflict by criticizing your partner's approach. Be glad he's a hands-on dad, even if you think he's handling the baby like a football: Babies benefit from male-style care.

4. You're arguing about money

WHAT'S BEHIND IT The costs associated with a new baby can add up quickly. And, if one of you is not returning to work, you're losing an income while gaining additional expenses. Fighting about money is the frequent result.

RELATIONSHIP SAVER Agree on a monthly budget before the baby is born; if you both honor it, you won't have to argue about spending, says Carrie Goghill Kuntz, a financial planner and co-founder of the D.B. Boot & Co. financial planning firm in Pittsburgh, Pa. Kuntz also recommends using a debit card for all your purchases; that way, if you can't afford something, you can't buy it.

5. You're becoming two ships passing in the night

WHAT'S BEHIND IT Each of you craves some time to yourself, so on weekends one of you cares for the baby in the morning and the other takes the afternoon shift. The result? You rarely see each other.

RELATIONSHIP SAVER Change your expectations, and instead of dates, think errands, Orbuch suggests. Go to the dog park or grocery store together, and take the baby with you—there's no need for a sitter and you'll share the care duties. Plus, you'll have fun introducing your baby to new experiences and places.

> ✳ Be glad he's a hands-on dad, even if you think he's handling the baby like a football: Babies benefit from male-style care.

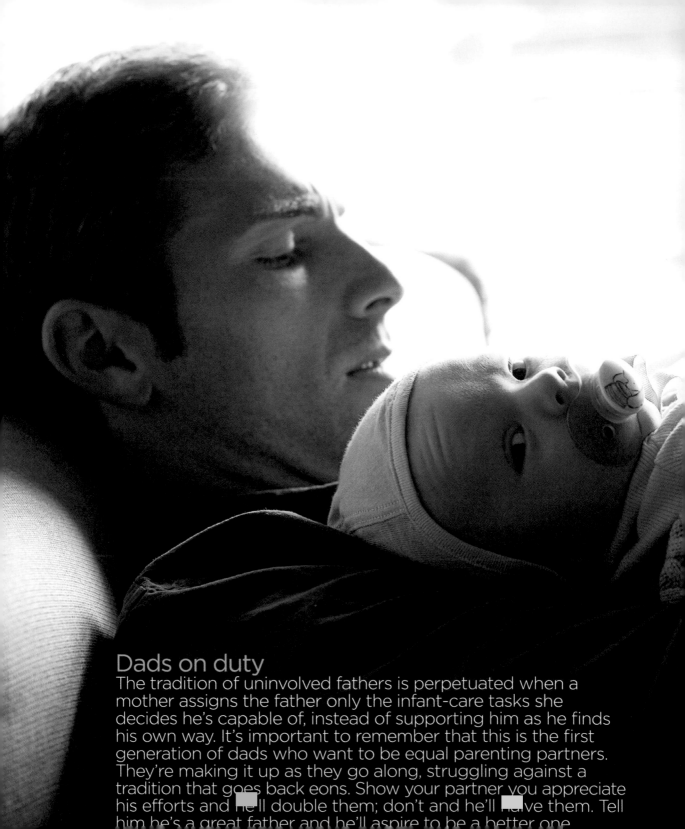

Dads on duty

The tradition of uninvolved fathers is perpetuated when a mother assigns the father only the infant-care tasks she decides he's capable of, instead of supporting him as he finds his own way. It's important to remember that this is the first generation of dads who want to be equal parenting partners. They're making it up as they go along, struggling against a tradition that goes back eons. Show your partner you appreciate his efforts and he'll double them; don't and he'll halve them. Tell him he's a great father and he'll aspire to be a better one.

Father knows best

When a man considers something really, really worth remembering, he writes it on his hand. Men don't use this memory jogger for non-life-threatening stuff, like anniversaries or e-mail addresses. No, palm-based crib notes are reserved for mission-critical info only. Like these 12 essential points of wisdom—culled from fathers who have been there and done that—which no new dad should ever, ever forget. If you write small, you'll be able to copy all of them onto your paws.

1. YOUR HOUSE IS TOO SMALL, it was always too small, and to suggest otherwise simply proves that your brain is too small.

2. YOU WILL BE SHORT ON CASH. You will not buy clothes for yourself for a year. You will consider canceling cable. You will never own a flat-screen TV. But there will always be money for a crib, three car seats, two strollers and more plastic things in DayGlo colors than you can throw a rattle at.

3. THERE WILL COME A DAY when you'll be your child's hero. Enjoy it—it won't last forever.

4. WHEN YOUR MOTHER PULLS YOU ASIDE and tells you that breastfeeding will ruin your wife's breasts, that babies only need to eat every four hours and that if you pick him up every time he cries he'll never be independent enough to go to summer camp, don't believe her.

5. YOUR CHILD WILL LIKE HER BEST for a long time. You'll get your turn—it just comes much later.

6. WHATEVER BAD PHASE YOUR KID IS GOING THROUGH, you'll find a solution. However, by the time you do that, he will be on to a new, even more confusing phase.

7. YOU'LL BE SURPRISED and amazed at how well you can function on so little sleep—and for how long.

8. YOU CAN'T TRADE IN those useless gifts for takeout.

9. THINGS YOU THOUGHT WOULD MAKE YOU SICK but don't: baby poop, baby pee and baby puke—and having all of them on your shirt at once.

10. YOU'LL GET MORE ADVICE from your childless friends. Parents will usually shrug and say, "It'll pass."

11. YOU CAN TASTE THE BREAST MILK, but you won't like it.

12. OF COURSE, IT CHANGES EVERYTHING. That's the whole point, isn't it?

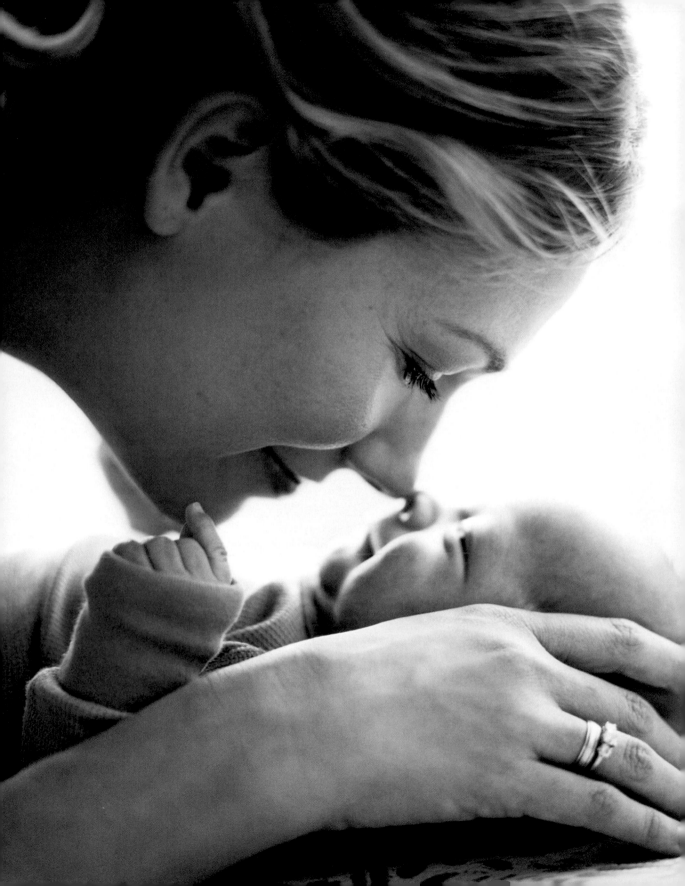

BONDING AND BREASTFEEDING | 5

Now that your baby has arrived, you may find

it's hard to tear yourself away from her. Or, you may not yet know how you feel about this new person in your life. Experts agree that the bonding process is different for everyone. But rest assured that each time you change a diaper, encourage her to smile or hold her close, you're building upon and deepening the mother-baby bond.

Looking for more ways to foster your brand new mommy-and-me relationship? Breastfeeding is good for both of you: Not only does it offer a chance for one-on-one time with your baby, it provides her with the nutrients she needs—and allows you to burn up to 500 calories a day! Plus, the following workouts help you get back in shape with your baby by your side. The best part? No babysitter required!

While you were pregnant, you undoubtedly found yourself dreamily obsessing about your baby or acting uncharacteristically absent-minded. If so, you actually may have been doing something very important: bonding with your baby. This detachment from worldly concerns is a lot like falling in love, and it's what leads to the emotional tie between parent and child.

But the common expectation that you must bond deeply with your baby instantly after he's born is unrealistic and can lead to anxiety if it doesn't happen that way. A little knowledge can help make things go more smoothly and put you at ease. So will knowing that the window of opportunity for bonding remains open longer than you might think.

Bonding: a natural process

Given the right conditions, bonding—or attachment— occurs naturally. "It will happen if the baby and mother are just left alone," says pediatrician William Sears, M.D., author of 2001's *The Attachment Parenting Book.* "Bonding is not something you have to plan for—like milk, it will flow." But Sears also says that a mother should not be worried if it doesn't happen immediately. "Bonding is not instant glue," he adds.

For most new moms, bonding takes time. "Attachment is a process that occurs over the first year of life as the relationship develops," explains Alison Steier, Ph.D., director of clinical training for Southwest Human Development's Harris Infant and Early Childhood Mental Health Training Institute in Phoenix. "It's the ongoing exchange between parent and child that creates the bond."

If you're concerned that you may not be bonding with your baby as quickly as you "should," consider that adoptive parents, who often are not present at their child's birth, are capable of bonding as closely as birth parents. It also helps to know that our physiology aids the process. "Every time you hold, nurse or otherwise take care of your baby," Sears explains, "you get a burst of oxytocin, which has been called the 'hormone of love.'" So talk and read to your baby, play with him face to face, and look into his eyes when you feed, bathe and dress him. Savor every moment together.

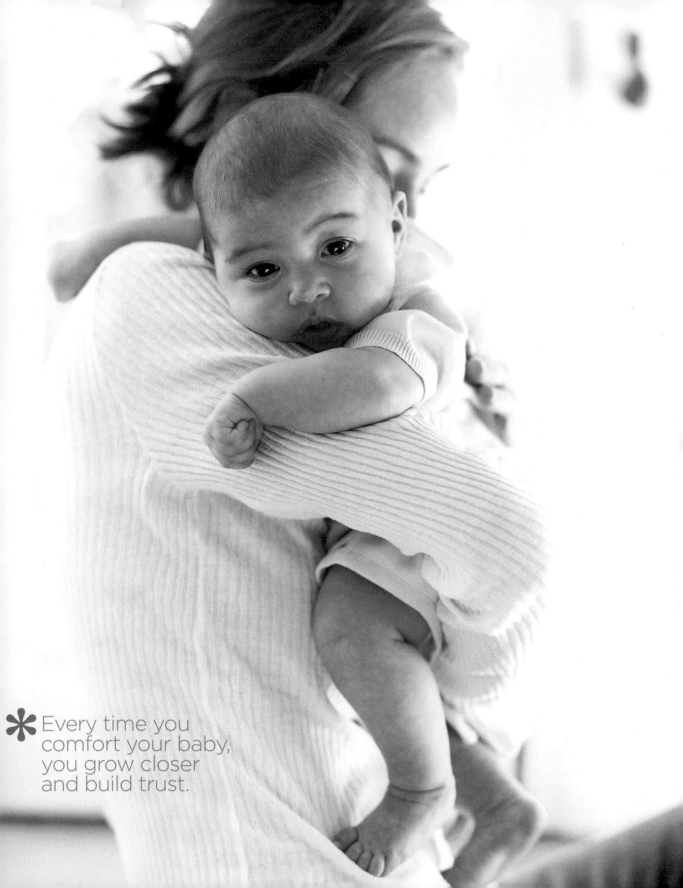

*Every time you comfort your baby, you grow closer and build trust.

Mommy-and-me yoga
Bond with your baby as you shape up with this gentle workout.

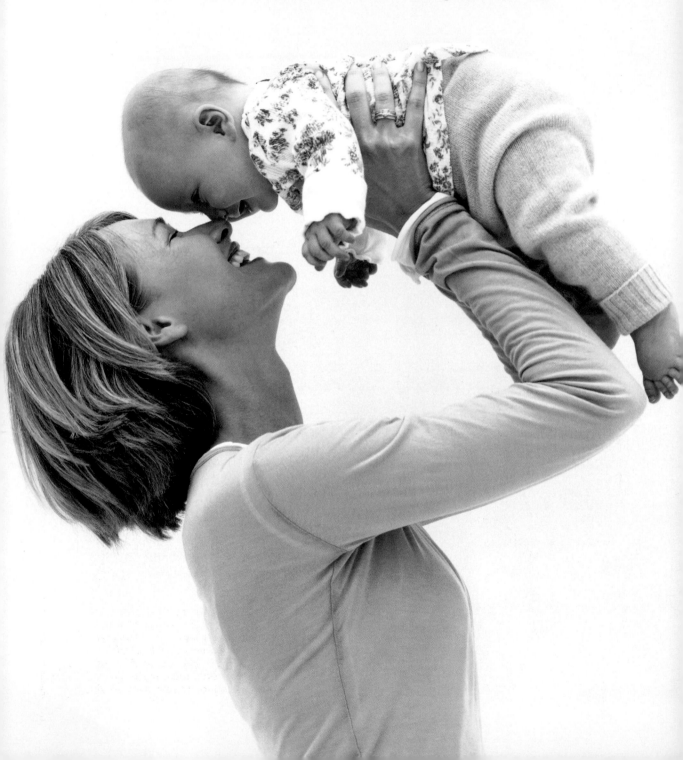

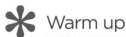 Warm up

UNION MEDITATION **Sit erect on a pillow in a comfortable, cross-legged position, cradling your baby close to your heart. Close your eyes and inhale deeply through your nose, filling your belly and expanding your ribs. Exhale deeply through your nose, feeling your belly draw in. Continue to breathe deeply as you feel the connection between you and your baby.**

"Yoga is union, breath, stillness and love," says Jo Ann Colker-Arison, a hatha yoga teacher in Los Angeles and creator of the postnatal DVD *Yoga Ma Baby Ga: Mama & Me Postnatal Yoga*. The following program focuses on the connection between mother and baby while strengthening the muscles most taxed during pregnancy and delivery.

Begin by trying one pose at a time, repeating for five full breaths and progressing to 10. If you feel any discomfort, stop and wait a few days before trying again. It's best to wait six weeks before starting any fitness program—longer if you had a Cesarean section—so check with your doctor first.

1

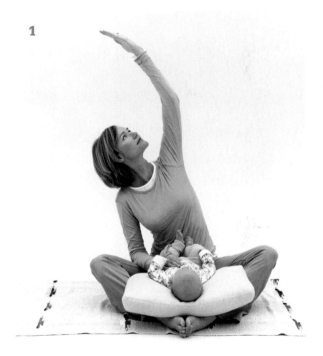

1 SOLE TO SOLE Sit on a pillow with the soles of your feet touching. Place your baby on a pillow or blanket, lying faceup between your legs. Keeping your right hand on your baby, sit up tall and draw your abs in. Inhale, then exhale as you lift your left arm up and lean to the right [shown]. Repeat on the other side. Then, inhale and exhale as you lean forward and round your spine, playing peekaboo with your baby.

✳ Do double duty: Strengthen your abdominals, arms, chest and shoulders while you spend time with your baby.

2

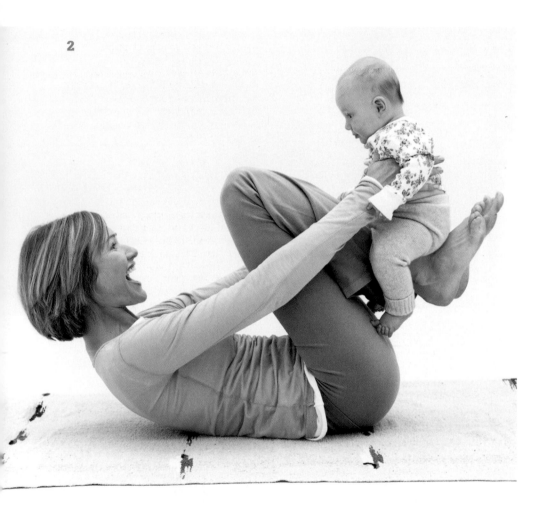

2

ROCK AND ROLL
Lie on your back on a comfortable surface, bring your knees close to your chest and hold your baby securely on your ankles or shins (depending on whether he can hold his head up). Exhale as you draw your belly in and lift your head and shoulders off the floor, bringing knees and baby closer to your chest as you make eye contact with him [shown]. Lower head and shoulders to starting position.

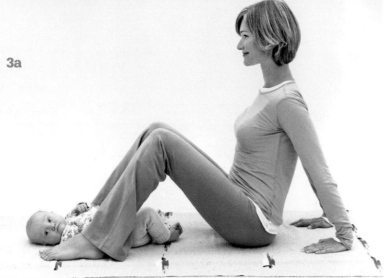

3a

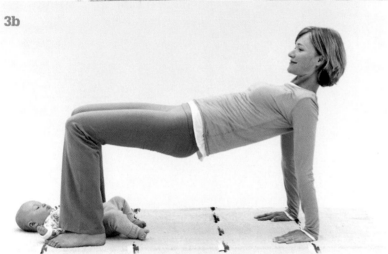

3b

3 REVERSE TABLETOP

Place your baby on a comfortable surface between your feet. Sit tall with your legs bent, palms down and behind hips, shoulders back and down, chest lifted [A]. Pressing into your hands and keeping shoulders back and down, inhale, then exhale as you lift your hips to a comfortable position keeping your neck relaxed [B]. Hold for 1 full breath, then lower hips to starting position.

4 SPHINX TO DOWN DOG

Lie on your belly, legs straight and slightly apart, your baby lying faceup. Place palms down, elbows under shoulders. Draw abs in and squeeze buttocks, shoulders back and down. Press into forearms to lift chest slightly [A]. Hold for 1 full breath, then bend legs, straighten arms and push back into Down Dog [B]. Hold for 1 breath, then bend legs and slowly lower onto belly.

4a

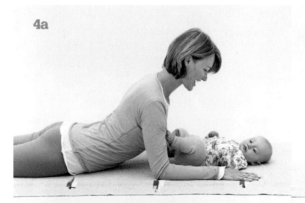

4b

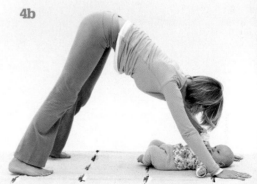

Bye-bye, baby fat

Make your baby a part of your exercise routine. It's good for you and fun for her.

The following strengthening moves can be done with your baby. Keep your abs drawn in and your shoulders back and down during each move. Be sure to cradle your baby's head securely, and don't forget to play and talk with her while you exercise. Wait six weeks before starting this workout and be sure to check with your doctor first.

1 BABY DANCING Holding your baby in your arms or in a front carrier, sway back and forth or dance the cha-cha [shown]. Keep your feet moving to gently raise your heart rate. Continue for 5 minutes, working up to 10.

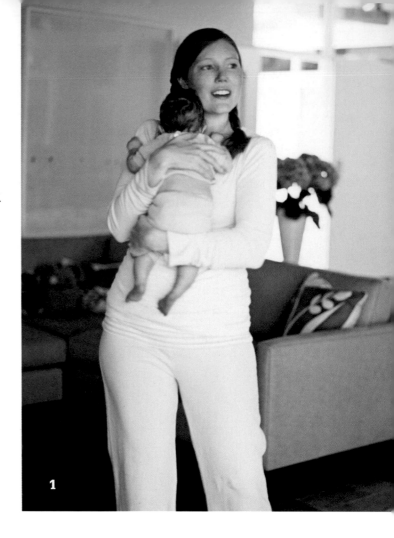

1

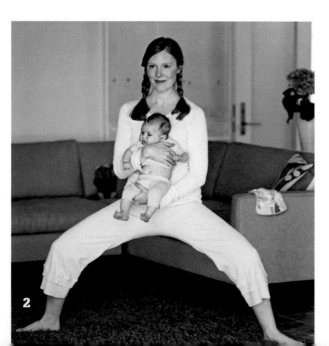

2

2

CRADLE PLIÉ
Holding your baby to your chest, stand with feet wider than hip distance, toes slightly turned out and abs tight. Keeping your pelvis still, bend your knees [shown]. Straighten your legs and squeeze your glutes (butt) as you return to starting position. Repeat 10 times, working up to 30.

3 **KISS THE BABY PUSH-UP** On your hands and knees, place your baby on her back, underneath your chest. With your wrists under your shoulders and your head in line with your spine, pull your abs in—your body should form a straight line from head to hips [shown]. Bend your elbows to lower your torso and give your baby a kiss. Push back up to starting position. Repeat 5 times, working up to 15.

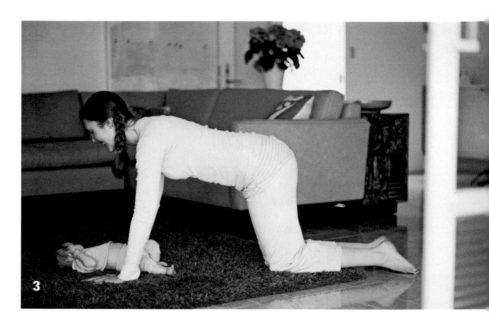

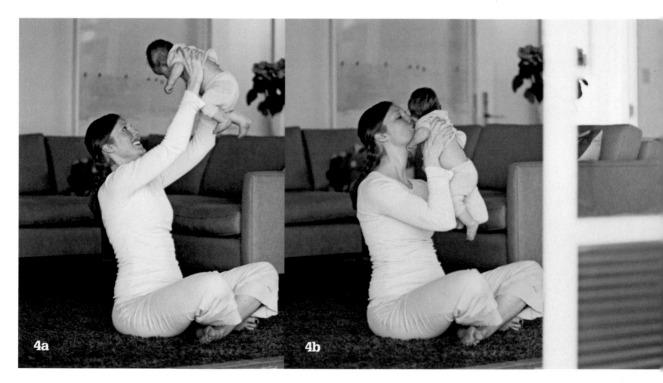

4 **BABY ELEVATORS** Sit with your knees bent and ankles crossed. Place your baby on your ankles facing you. Maintaining a straight back, gently lift her toward the ceiling, keeping your elbows slightly bent [A]. Slowly lower your baby toward your chest and give her a kiss [B]. Push her back up into the air. Repeat 5 times, working up to 15.

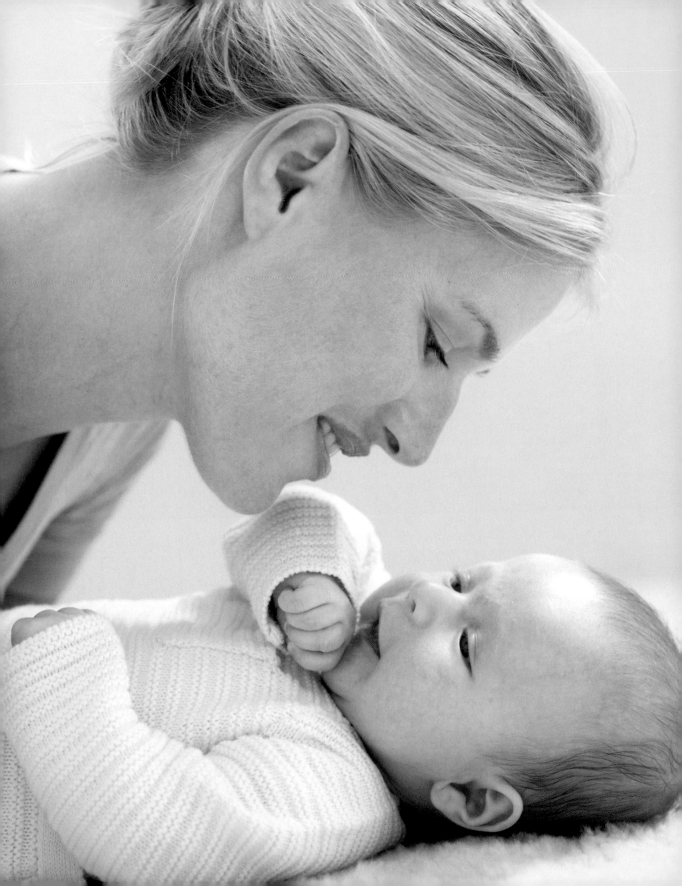

Tummy time

Tone your abs with your baby by your side.

As a new mom, you don't have to choose between spending time with your baby and getting rid of that postpartum belly.

"Working out with your baby creates a bonding experience between you and establishes a foundation for lifelong healthy habits," says Mary Beth Knight, creator of the *MommyMuscle Restore The Core* DVD. "This workout incorporates learning and stimulation for your baby through ball play, singing and counting, while giving you a challenging workout right at home." The moves are designed to help get rid of the "pooch" that pregnancy leaves behind by focusing on the deep abdominal muscles.

You can do this workout every other day, but wait six weeks before starting; longer if you've had a Cesarean section. Check with your doctor before beginning this or any exercise program.

✳ Warm up

Put on your favorite music, pick up your baby and dance around the room for five minutes.

What you need

A mat or blanket big enough for you and your baby, as well as a small, soft ball. During the workout, interact with your baby by singing, counting or playing with the ball as you do the moves. Repeat each move 4 times, working up to 10.

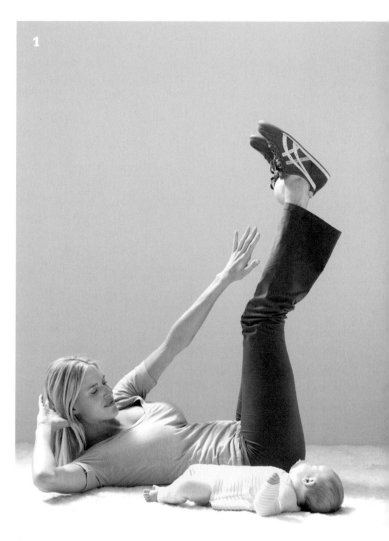

1 **CROSS AND REACH** Lie on your back with your baby beside you. Holding a small, soft ball between your feet, extend your legs to the ceiling. Raise your left arm above your head. Inhale, then exhale as you reach your left hand toward your right ankle, lifting your shoulder off the mat [shown]. Counting or singing to your baby (babies love to hear your voice!), hold for 10 seconds, working up to 15. Switch sides and repeat.

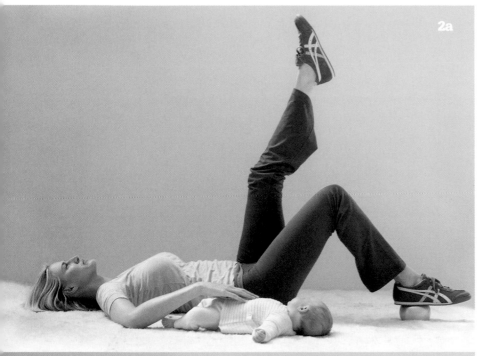

2a

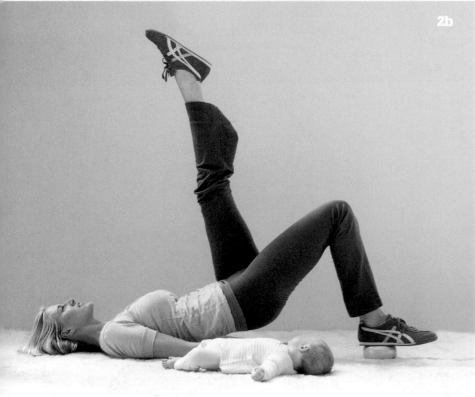

2b

2

SINGLE-LEG BRIDGE
Lie on your back with knees bent, feet flat and your baby beside you. Place the ball under your right foot and press your arms into the floor, palms down, for balance. Extend your left leg up to the ceiling [A]. Inhale, then exhale as you press into the ball with your right foot, lifting your hips into a bridge position [B]. Inhale as you lower your hips towards the floor. Do 4 to 10 times. Switch ball to the other foot and repeat.

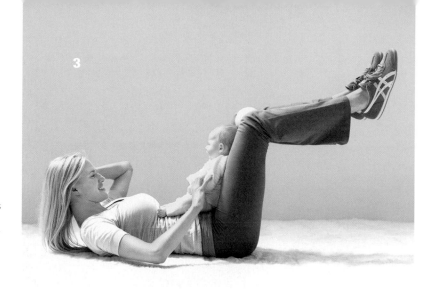

3 TABLETOP WITH BALL SQUEEZE

Lie on your back with your knees bent in a tabletop position and your baby propped against your thighs. Squeeze the ball between your knees, placing one hand behind your head and one hand on your baby to steady him. Inhale, then exhale as you draw your abs in and lift your head and shoulders off the floor, looking at your baby [shown]. Hold for 10 seconds, working up to 15. Lower head and repeat.

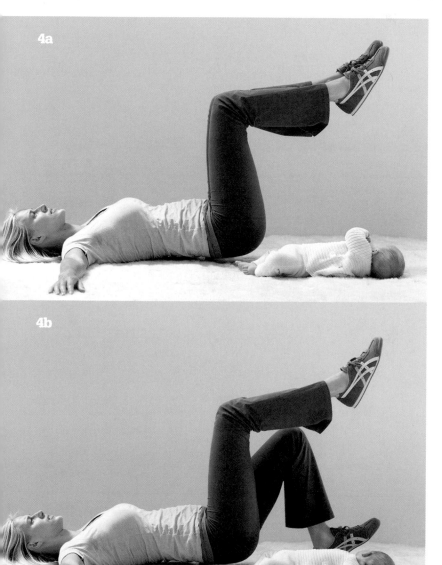

4

TABLETOP ENERGIZED

Lie on your back with your baby beside you. Place the ball under your lower back, just below your waist. Move your arms into a T-position, palms down. Take a moment to find your balance, then raise your legs to a tabletop position, toes pointed [A]. Inhale and drop your left heel toward the floor [B]. Exhale and bring the heel back up. Do 5 times, then switch sides.

Cool down

Lie on your back with your baby at your side. To stretch your lower back, hug your knees into your chest and rock from side to side. Breathe deeply and pause at each side for 10 to 30 seconds. Sit up and take a moment to breathe slowly, while holding your baby.

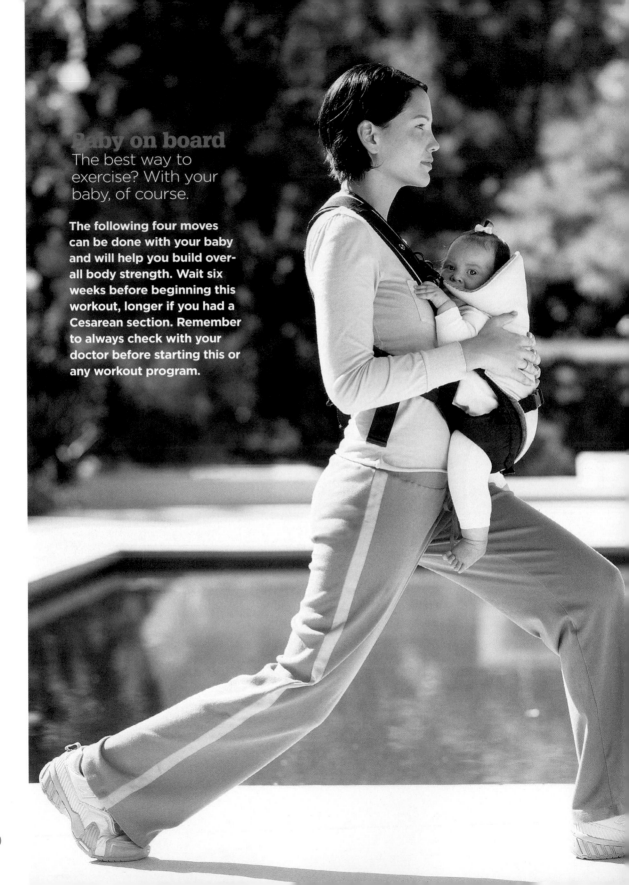

Baby on board
The best way to exercise? With your baby, of course.

The following four moves can be done with your baby and will help you build over-all body strength. Wait six weeks before beginning this workout, longer if you had a Cesarean section. Remember to always check with your doctor before starting this or any workout program.

✻ For a cardio boost, walk with your baby in a front carrier or sling; she will make your workouts more effective as she grows. Walk 20 to 30 minutes, three to five times a week.

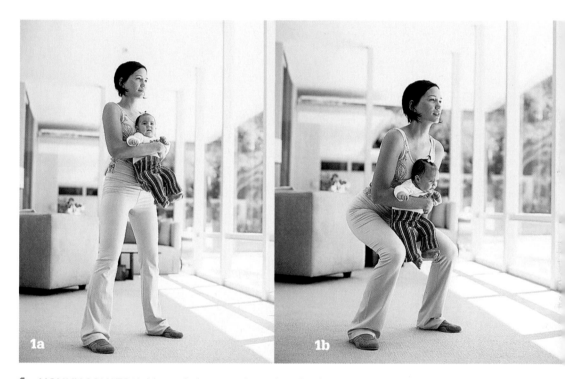

1a 1b

1 **MOMMY SQUATS** Hold your baby securely at chest level. Stand with your feet hip-width apart, your knees slightly bent and abs tight [A]. Bend your knees, bringing your thighs as close to parallel to the floor as possible, keeping knees behind toes [B]. Rise slowly without locking knees. Repeat for 3 minutes, about 20 to 25 reps.

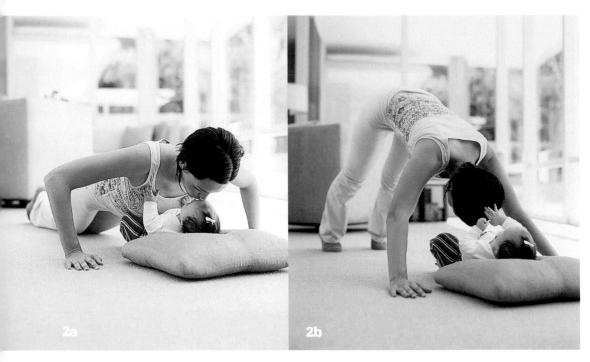

2a

2b

2 INVERTED V PUSH-UP KISS Get down on your hands and knees. Place your baby faceup on a large pillow under your chest. With your hands wider than your shoulders, ab muscles contracted and neck straight, bend your elbows to lower your chest toward your baby; give her a kiss [A]. Slowly straighten your arms and legs as you press your hips toward the ceiling to form an inverted V [B]. Slowly lower to starting position. Repeat for 3 minutes, about 20 to 25 reps.

3 REVERSE-CURL PEEKABOO
Lie faceup and bring your knees toward your chest. Place your baby's chest on your shins [A]. Holding her there, contract your abs to gently tilt your hips up off the floor as you lift your head, neck and shoulders to play peekaboo [B]. Lower and repeat. Repeat for 2 minutes, about 20 to 25 reps.

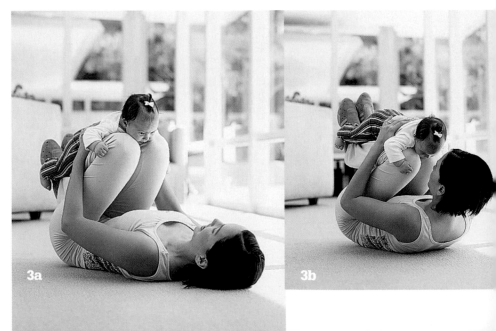

3a

3b

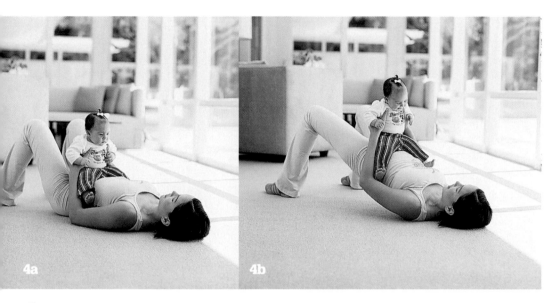

4a

4b

4 BABY BRIDGE Lie faceup, knees bent, feet flat on the floor and parallel, ankles under knees. Place your baby on your hips, just below your bellybutton, and hold her securely [A]. Keeping your head on the floor, lift your hips to form a straight line from shoulders to knees. Pause at the top, squeezing buttocks and thighs, pressing into heels [B]. Slowly lower to starting position. Repeat for 2 minutes, about 20 to 25 reps. Strengthens thighs and buttocks.

Exercise and breastfeeding help prevent baby blues

Scientists have discovered that systemic inflammation is a risk factor for depression and that stress increases inflammation. This helps explain post-partum depression, says Kathleen Kendall-Tackett, Ph.D., research associate at the Family Research Laboratory, University of New Hampshire in Durham. The body produces higher levels of pro-inflammatory chemicals during the last trimester of pregnancy to protect against infection and prepare for labor. The stresses of new motherhood, including disturbed sleep, fatigue and postpartum pain, also boost the chemicals' production, even when the mother isn't suffering from emotional stress.

But two simple, drug-free activities—exercise and breastfeeding—can help. "Exercise keeps the chemical cascade of stress hormones and inflammation from happening," says Kendall-Tackett. "People with better physical fitness have lower inflammation responses to stress, so there is a short- and long-term advantage to exercising. And when nursing is going well, feeding the baby at the breast buffers stress for about 30 minutes." Kendall-Tackett notes that pediatric experts recommend breastfeeding for at least a year. "Moms will get the anti-stress/anti-inflammatory response for as long as they nurse," she says.

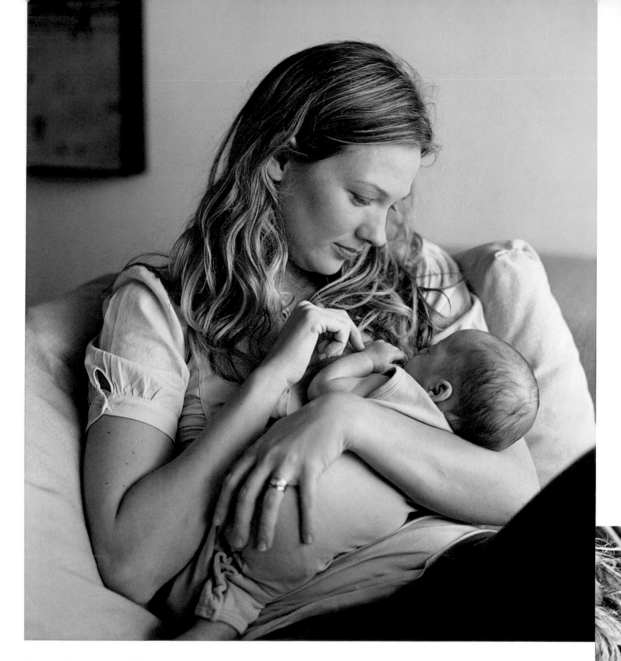

Ready, set, flow

Experts agree: Nursing your baby is one of the best things you can do for him. But good things don't always come easily. Marathon feeding sessions, engorged breasts and sore nipples are some of the challenges you might face as a nursing mom, especially in the beginning. Fortunately, the majority of problems can be overcome with information and practice, says Sue Tiller, R.N., an international board-certified lactation consultant in Centreville, Va., and the author of 2005's *Breastfeeding 101: A Step-by-Step Guide To Successfully Nursing Your Baby.*

From how to position your little one at the breast to the best time for introducing a bottle, here are the six most important steps to successful breastfeeding.

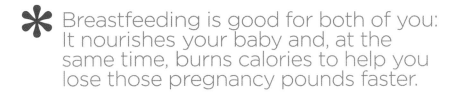

*Breastfeeding is good for both of you: It nourishes your baby and, at the same time, burns calories to help you lose those pregnancy pounds faster.

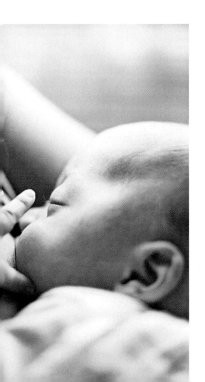

1. HOP TO IT. After a vaginal delivery, as long as there are no complications, try to nurse right away. If you've had a Cesarean section, you may have to wait until surgery is complete—but try to breastfeed within the first hour.

Don't stress if your baby doesn't suckle at first; babies born at term have stores of calories and fluid that make it unnecessary for them to eat much early on. So unless she's a preemie, she shouldn't need much nourishment for the first few days of her life.

2. MAKE SURE YOU'RE COMFY. Once your baby is latched onto your breast and nursing, you won't want to interrupt her because you're uncomfortable. So take a minute to settle into a comfortable, relaxed position before starting to breastfeed, advises Terriann Shell, an international board-certified lactation consultant in Big Lake, Alaska.

When you're just starting out, sit up straight in an armchair. Lay a firm pillow across your lap so your baby is level with your breast, and prop up your elbows on the chair arms or pillows. Also put a pillow behind your back for support, if needed. Place your feet on a foot stool to bring your baby closer and help prevent back and arm strain.

3. LEARN THE CORRECT LATCH. A good latch (aka latch-on) is essential for your milk to flow properly and to keep your little piranha from making fish food of your nipples. (For a how-to, see "How to Get the Right Latch," pgs. 138-139.)

Breast milk is brimming with nutrients and antibodies that boost your newborn's immunity, aid digestion and promote brain development. An added bonus: Breastfeeding burns calories like crazy, helping you lose those pregnancy pounds faster. And it reduces your lifetime risk of developing breast or ovarian cancer and postmenopausal osteoporosis.

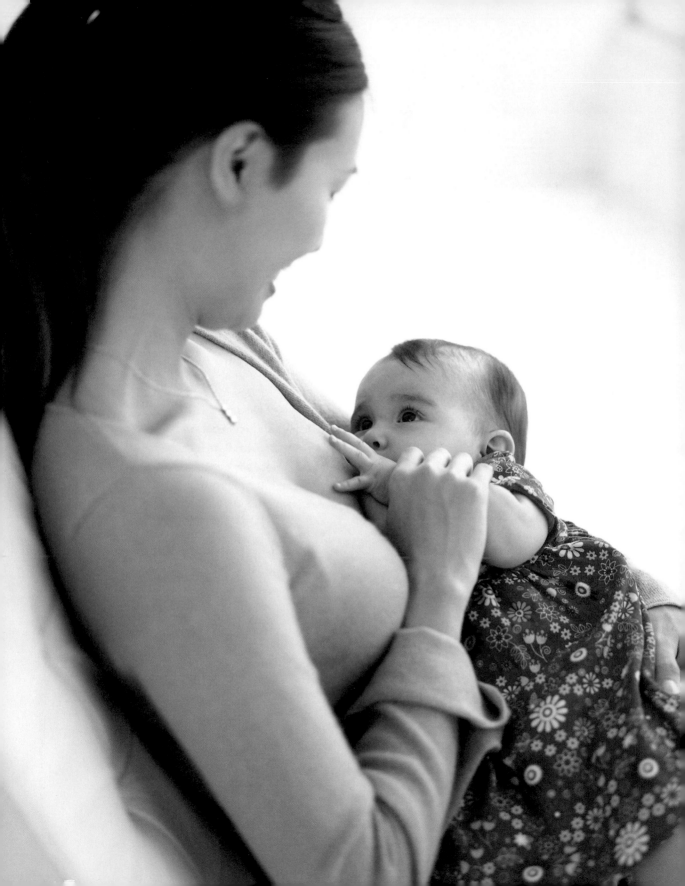

Breast milk is brimming with nutrients and antibodies that boost your newborn's immunity, aid digestion and promote brain development.

4. LET YOUR BABY GRAZE. Frequent and effective nursing is key to boosting your milk supply and ensuring your baby gets enough to eat. You should aim for at least eight to 12 feedings daily—about every two to three hours—for the first few weeks, says pediatrician Jane Morton, M.D., of Burgess Pediatrics in Menlo Park, Calif. At first, each nursing session could last anywhere from 20 to 45 minutes; as your milk production increases and your baby gets better at suckling, it shouldn't take as long. The number of feedings will also decrease.

In the first few weeks, when your baby is more sleepy than hungry, you may have to initiate many of these feedings—even if it means waking her. If she falls asleep within minutes of latching on, you can try rousing her by changing her diaper or undressing her.

5. HOLD OFF ON BOTTLES. While you may love the idea of pumping some milk and letting your partner take over a midnight feeding, wait to introduce a bottle for a month or so, until nursing is well established. Since it's easier to extract milk from an artificial nipple, giving a bottle too early could cause your baby to reject the breast in favor of the bottle's faster flow. But don't wait too long, either. "Babies tend to be open-minded at about 4 weeks of age," Morton says. "If you wait much longer, you may have trouble getting her to take a bottle."

6. DON'T GO IT ALONE. New moms who get plenty of guidance tend to breastfeed longer than those who don't. The best time to seek help? Before you need it. While you're in the hospital, spend time with the lactation consultant on staff. If your hospital doesn't have such an expert on-site, your nurse or pediatrician may be able to help.

After heading home, attend a breastfeeding support group (offered through some hospitals and La Leche League International: llli.org). In addition, the International Lactation Consultant Association (ilca.org) can provide valuable information or help you find a board-certified lactation consultant in your area.

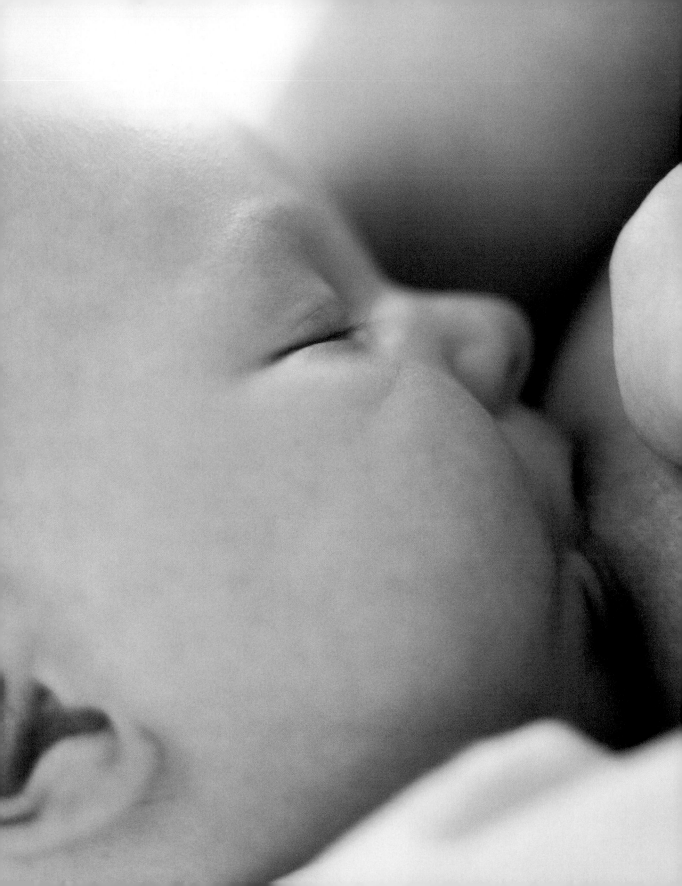

How to get the right latch

POSITION YOUR BABY ON HER SIDE so she is directly facing you, with her belly touching yours. Next, if necessary, prop up your baby with a pillow so her mouth is near your nipple, and hold her up to your breast; don't lean over toward her. If you've had a Cesarean section, place your baby on her back on a pillow close to your side. Her head should be next to your breast, with the rest of her body alongside you. Resting your arm on the pillow, support your baby's head with your hand and bring her mouth up to your breast (she will be tucked under your arm).

1. PLACE YOUR THUMB AND FINGERS around the outside of your areola (the dark area surrounding the nipple).

2. TILT YOUR BABY'S HEAD BACK SLIGHTLY and tickle her lips with your nipple until she opens her mouth wide. Be patient; this can take some time.

3. HELP HER "SCOOP" as much of your breast as possible into her mouth by placing her lower jaw on first, at the edge of the areola and well below the nipple.

4. TILT HER HEAD FORWARD, placing her upper jaw deeply on your breast. Make sure she takes the entire nipple and at least 1½ inches of the areola in her mouth. When the baby first latches on, you may feel intense, sometimes painful twinges that last a few seconds. But if the discomfort subsides within a minute or two, you'll know your baby is properly positioned on your breast.

1

2

3

4

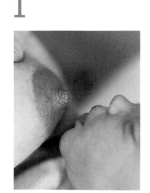
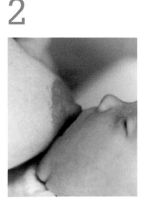
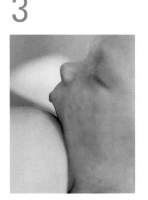
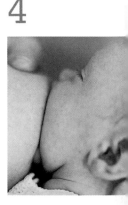

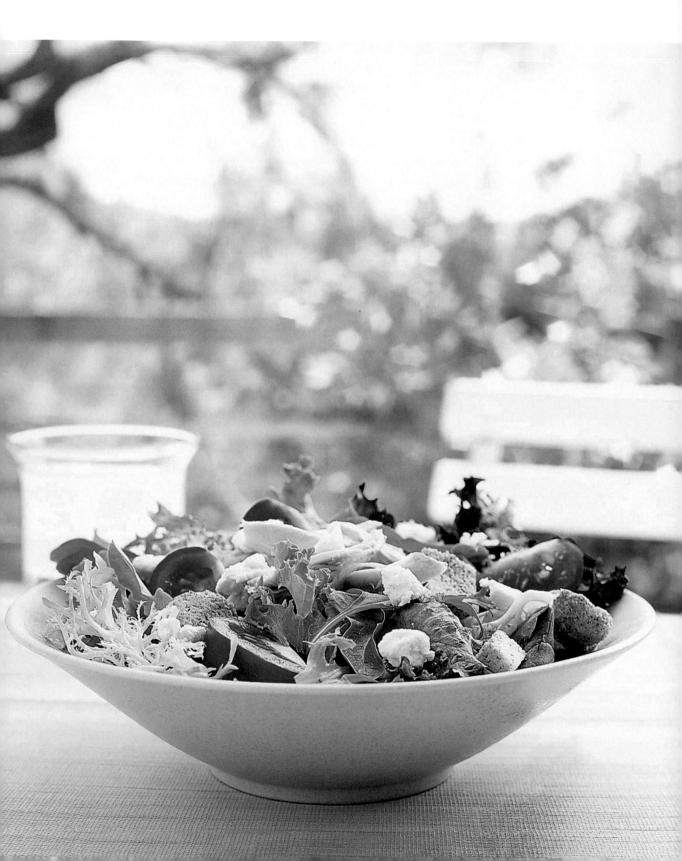

Still eating for two

It's important to make good nutrition a priority, especially if you're breastfeeding—after all, your baby is relying on you to supply all the nutrients he needs. We're here to help, with tasty tips and a one-day meal plan that will give you maximum nutrition with minimal effort.

AIM FOR THE A Your need for vitamin A skyrockets when you're nursing—from 770 micrograms a day during pregnancy to 1,300 when breastfeeding. Colorful, fresh fruits and vegetables are your best bets.
GET YOUR DAILY QUOTA 1 medium sweet potato and 1 cup vegetable juice.

GO FOR COLOR As a nursing mom, you need 120 milligrams (mg) of vitamin C every day. Eating plenty of colorful fruits and vegetables will help you reach this amount.
GET YOUR DAILY QUOTA 1 cup orange juice, 1 ½ cups sliced strawberries or 1 ½ cups broccoli.

BONE UP ON CALCIUM Your calcium needs are the same before, during and after pregnancy: 1,000 milligrams (mg) per day. But since many women don't meet the minimum, it's critical to consume calcium rich foods such as dairy (e.g., low-fat cheese, yogurt and milk), calcium-fortified soy milk, calcium-fortified juices and cereals, and dark leafy greens.
GET YOUR DAILY QUOTA 1 cup nonfat yogurt, 2 glasses low-fat (1%) milk and 1 slice cheese.

FOCUS ON FOLATE Getting enough folate—500 micrograms (mcg) daily if you're nursing—from diet alone can be difficult, but eating plenty of dried beans, grains and fortified foods (such as cereals and breads) will make it easier.
GET YOUR DAILY QUOTA 1 cup fortified raisen bran cereal, ½ cup cooked pinto beans, ½ cup spinach, 1 cup orange juice and 1 slice whole-wheat bread.

EAT YOUR MEAT (OR TOFU) Your protein requirement stays the same during pregnancy and while breastfeeding: 71 grams per day. Sources include dairy, meat, poultry, fish, tofu, dried beans and whole grains.

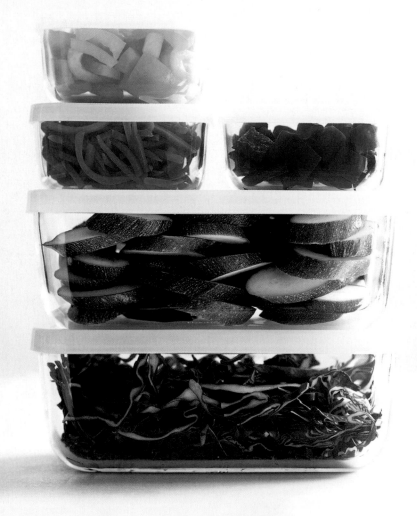

✳ Fruits and vegetables are a good source of vitamin C and the more colorful your choices, the better.

GET YOUR DAILY QUOTA 2 eggs, 3 ounces roast beef, 2 cups low-fat (1%) milk, 4 ounces cooked salmon and 2 slices whole-wheat bread.

DRINK UP Breast milk is 87 percent water, so be sure to load up on fluids. Water and milk are your best bets; if you drink caffeinated coffee, try to limit it to one to three 8-ounce cups a day. As for sodas, limit them to one or two a day, and opt for diet, caffeine-free varieties.
GET YOUR DAILY QUOTA Eight 8-ounce glasses of fluids, even more if you are thirsty or are exercising.

One-day menu for nursing moms

This quick, simple menu also is great for moms who aren't breastfeeding. But if you aren't burning those extra calories by nursing, be sure to forgo some items or you'll gain weight.

Breakfast

OATMEAL WITH WALNUTS & DATES
1½ cups cooked oatmeal mixed with
   1 tablespoon chopped walnuts,
   2 tablespoons chopped dates and
   2 teaspoons maple syrup
1 cup calcium-fortified orange juice
1 cup low-fat (2%) milk

Snack

BANANA & PEANUT BUTTER ON A BAGEL
1 banana
½ whole-grain bagel topped with 1 tablespoon
   crunchy peanut butter

Lunch

TUNA SALAD ON WHOLE-WHEAT BREAD
Dijon Tuna Sandwich: 6 ounces water-packed
   tuna, drained and mixed with 1 tablespoon
   mayonnaise, 2 teaspoons Dijon mustard
   and 1/4 cup shredded carrots, spread on two
   slices whole-wheat bread.
Side dish:
1½ cups bell pepper strips (mixed colors)
1 kiwi fruit

Snack

OATMEAL COOKIE & YOGURT
1 oatmeal raisin cookie
1 cup light vanilla yogurt

Dinner

TURKEY CHEESEBURGER & SALAD
Turkey & Swiss Burger: 4 ounces ground
   turkey, grilled or broiled and served on
   1 mixed-grain hamburger bun with a
   1-ounce slice Swiss cheese, 2 pieces leaf
   lettuce and 2 slices tomato.
1 baked sweet potato topped with 2
   teaspoons butter
Salad:
2 cups mixed greens (baby spinach,
   romaine, escarole and red-leaf lettuce)
   topped with 2 slices red onion, 1/4 cup
   chopped cucumber and 6 cherry
   tomatoes, 2 tablespoons balsamic
   vinaigrette dressing

Dessert

ICE CREAM AND STRAWBERRIES
½ cup dulce de leche ice cream served
   with ½ cup fresh sliced strawberries

NUTRITIONAL INFORMATION: 2,652 calories, 31% fat (92 g), 10% saturated fat (28 g), 50% carbohydrate (336 g), 19% protein (129 g), 40 g dietary fiber, 18 mg iron, 1,783 mg calcium, 5,077 mcg vitamin A, 496 mg vitamin C, 605 mcg folate, 16 mg zinc.

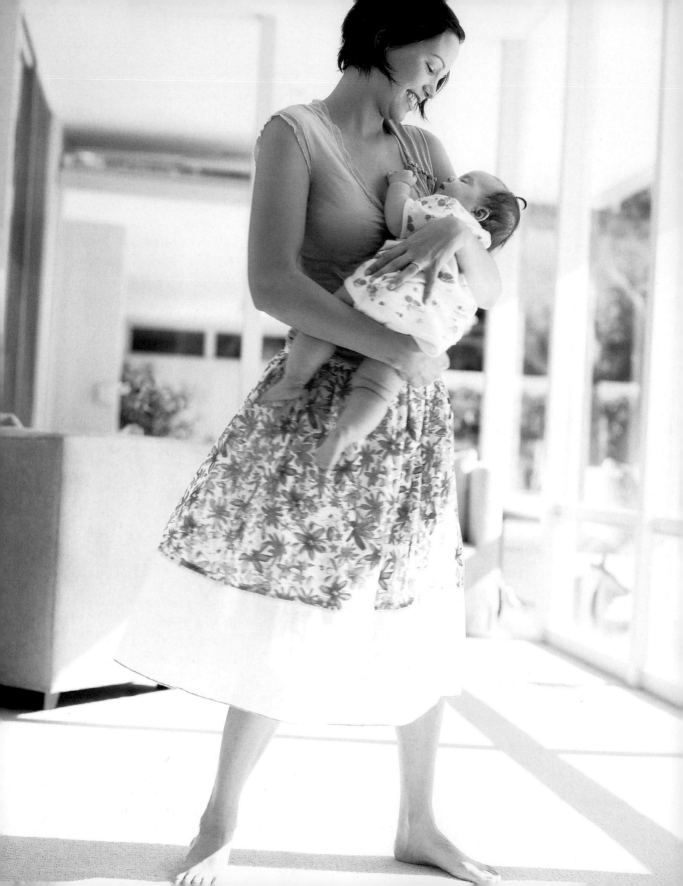

Play with me

What better way to bond with your baby than through play? Whether he's 9 weeks or 9 months old, your baby is guaranteed to be tickled pink by these developmental games.

NEWBORN TO 3 MONTHS | WHERE'S MOMMY?

Newborns have an innate fascination with voices, but they're not able to locate the source of a sound. To help your little one fine-tune this sense and also learn that his family provides laughter and smiles, place him in the middle of a bed or in an infant seat or hold him in your arms; get close to his face and talk or sing to him. Walk back and forth in front of him as you continue to talk and sing.

DEVELOPMENTAL SKILLS: listening; visual and social development; sensory exploration.

3 TO 6 MONTHS | AIRPLANE BABY

Help comfort your cranky baby—or simply have fun together—with this classic game. To start, hold him under his chest and belly, tummy down. (Be sure to support his neck if he doesn't yet have head control.) Swing him gently back and forth. Sing a song while you swing, too.

DEVELOPMENTAL SKILLS: upper-body strength; tactile stimulation; trust.

6 TO 9 MONTHS | KNEE RIDES

Once your baby has good head control, prop her up on your knees and gently bounce her as you babble or sing. Babbling supports her early efforts to communicate with sounds other than crying. When she says, "aahh," say, "aahh" in return; when she says, "goo," nod and say, "goo" back. Then try stretching out the words and adding to them ("ooh" becomes "ooooh-wah!").

DEVELOPMENTAL SKILLS: listening; language and social development; sensory exploration.

9 TO 12 MONTHS | PEEKABOO!

Peekaboo is a classic favorite with babies: First mommy's there, then mommy's gone, and then she's back again. Sometime around 6 or 7 months, babies start to understand that objects continue to exist even if they can't see them.

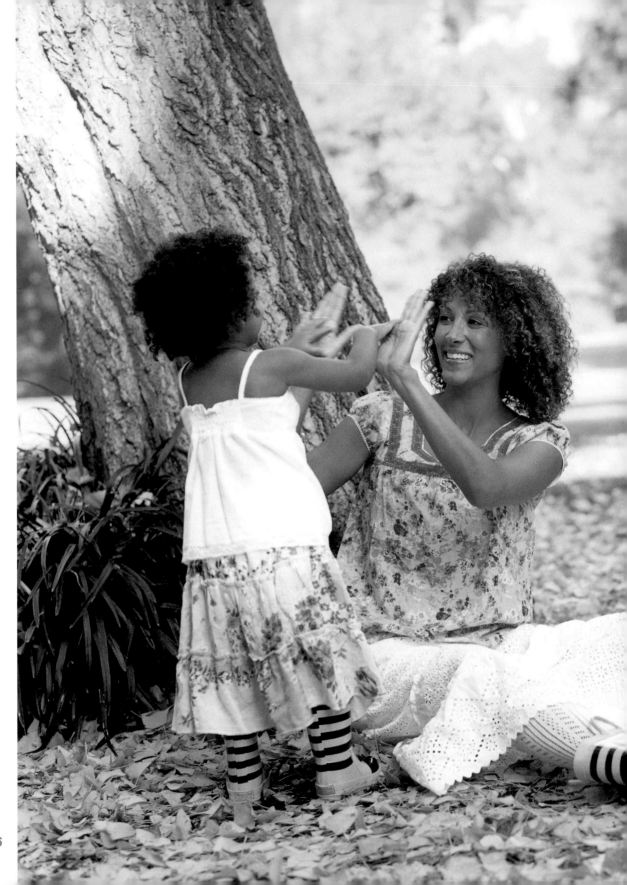

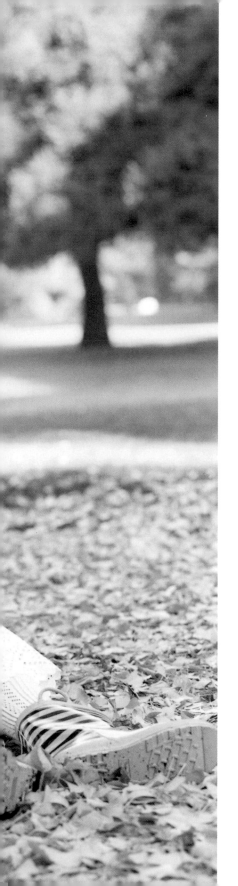

✳ Playing and singing with your baby are easy ways to foster bonding—and, share a laugh together, too!

Use your hands or hold a blanket or towel in front of your face, whisk it away and call, "Peekaboo!"
DEVELOPMENTAL SKILLS: object permanence; sensory exploration; social development.

12 TO 18 MONTHS | BUBBLES FOR BABY
Watching bubbles float through the air helps your baby practice her visual skills. Trying to swat at them is excellent practice for budding eye-hand coordination. Aiming large bubbles at a blanket or carpet gives older babies a chance to catch them. Bubbles outside are especially enchanting; blow them low to the ground so they drift skyward.
DEVELOPMENTAL SKILLS: cause-and-effect; eye-hand coordination; visual development.

18 TO 24 MONTHS | I'M GONNA GET YOU!
Babies love to be chased and surprised. Start crawling or running after your baby, saying, "I'm gonna get you!" Then gently grab him and say, "I got you!" Lift him up in the air, kiss his neck and tickle his ribs, but keep it gentle. A good game of chase will keep him on his toes as a toddler (and, give you a workout, too) and evolve into classic big-kids games such as hide-and-seek and tag.
DEVELOPMENTAL SKILLS: gross-motor skills; social development; balance; trust.

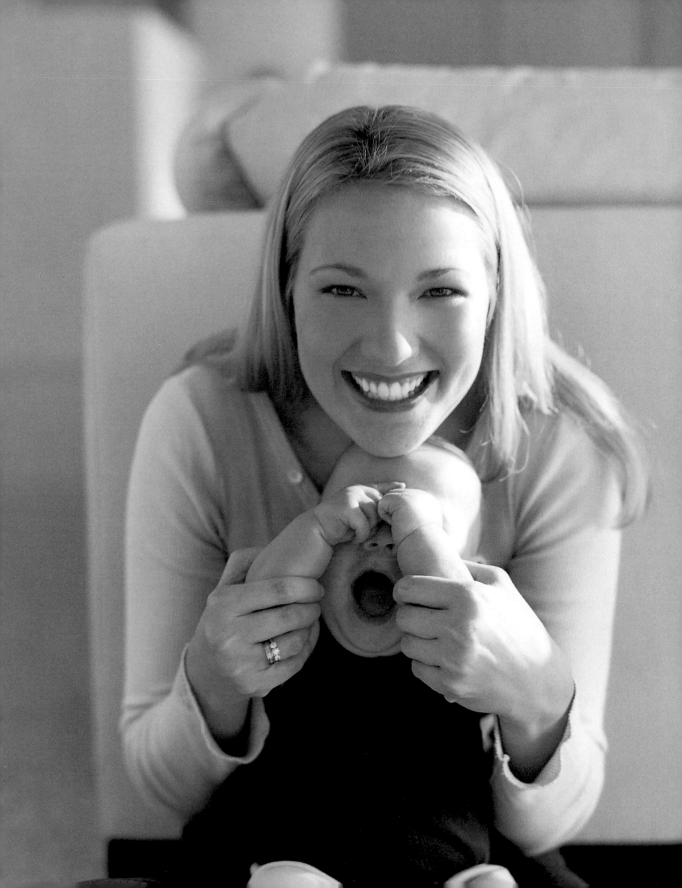

BECOMING A CONFIDENT MOM | 6

Caring for a new baby can make even the most self-assured individual doubtful: Am I swaddling correctly? Is he too hot in that sweater? How will I ever learn to clip such tiny nails? The following 10 tips will help you become a more confident mom—from the best ways to handle bad advice to banishing the guilt. What's more, those women returning to work often struggle with trying to balance being a mom and a professional. Our advice? Stop worrying. You're a better employee and mother than you think.

Whether you stay at home, work part time or 9-to-5, it's vital to carve out time for yourself. Go for a run, find a cozy reading nook free from distractions or meet up with a friend for a cup of coffee and conversation. It's important to nurture yourself both physically and mentally—because a happy mom means a happy baby.

Being a mom is largely a self-confidence game. But while gaining confidence is important to becoming a mom, being unsure isn't all bad. "If uncertain feelings are creeping in, it shows you're taking your job as a mom with a lot of responsibility," says Yvonne Thomas, Ph.D., a licensed psychologist in Los Angeles. "By recognizing the effect you have on shaping your child's personality, self-esteem and physical well-being, you're taking the first step toward being a great mother."

Your baby already thinks you're pretty top-notch. The following 10 tips will help you believe it, too.

1. ACT LIKE A BABY-CARE PRO. To be more self-confident, begin by acting like you are. Your baby will feel safer, calmer and happier, and soon assuredness won't be a guise as you get the hang of clipping tiny nails or giving a bath. "Take a cue from kindergarten teachers," says Frances Xavier Reis, M.D., a pediatrician at Talbert Medical Group in Downey, Calif. "Speak lower and slower to calm both you and your baby down." (For more tips, see our bonus chapter on baby-care basics, pgs. 170-176.)

2. DON'T CAVE IN TO BAD ADVICE. Don't relent when barraged with suggestions from people who act as if they know more than you do. Instead, call your pediatrician. It never hurts to double check on advice you're unsure of or uncomfortable with. Plus, it will ease your mind knowing you have the correct information from a source you trust— your child's doctor.

3. LOSE THE AUDIENCE. When your baby is hard to calm, find a place to work it out in private. Not only will this get your child out of an overstimulating environment, but it also will protect you from unsolicited advice. If relatives try to follow you, go into the bathroom and shut the door. Then turn on the fan—the white noise may do the trick. For both of you.

4. OVERCOME "BAD MOMMY" SYNDROME. All moms feel inadequate at some point. When you feel the guilt coming on, follow these guidelines: First, put your offense in perspective. Did you lock her in the closet or leave her in a hot,

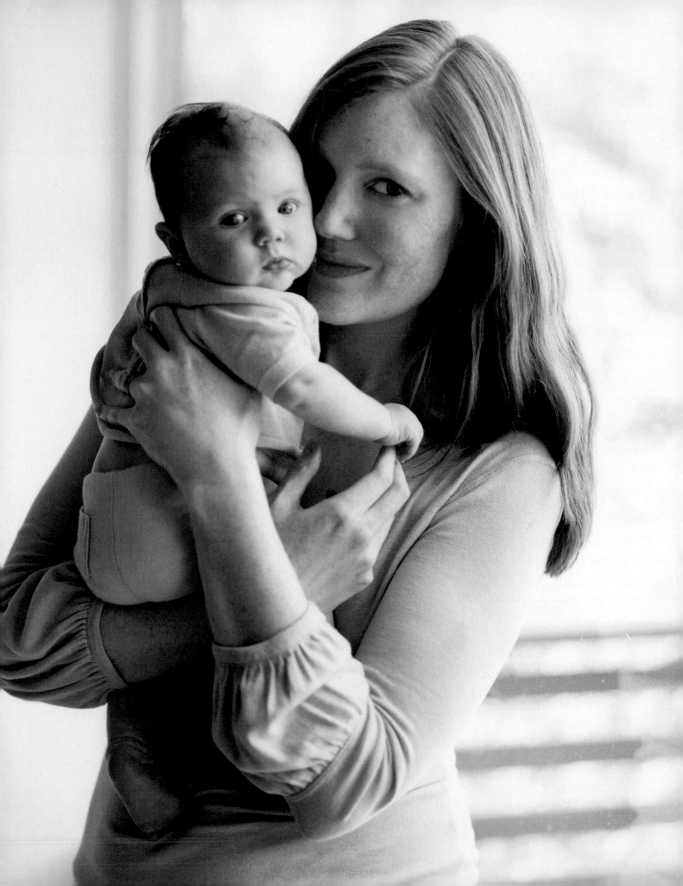

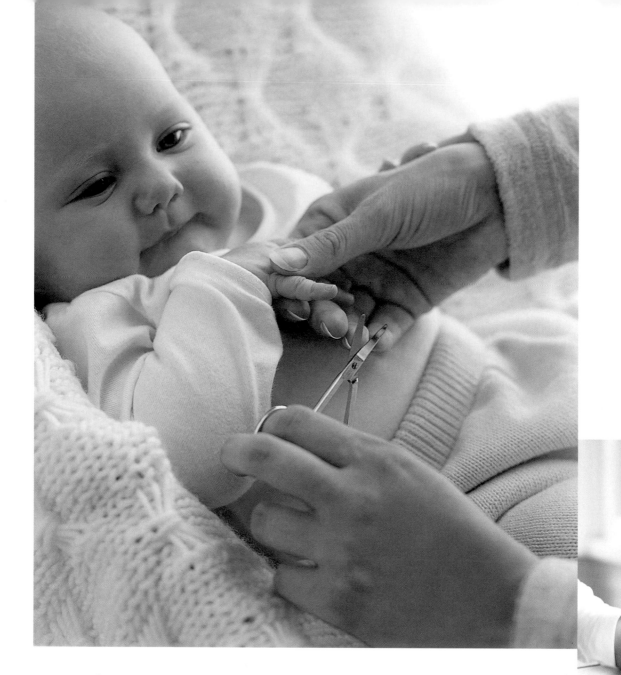

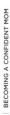

✳ Clipping tiny nails or bathing your baby may seem daunting at first. But, the more you do it, the easier it becomes.

parked car? Of course not. Second, remind your too-critical inner voice that all children—even babies—get hurt sometimes. If yours doesn't, you're probably being overprotective. Third, make a change that will prevent the problem—and guilt—next time. (e.g., If your baby is learning to sit and falls, a supportive pillow may mitigate future topples.) Finally, put the incident where it belongs: in the past.

5. BE DECISIVE. Tune into your gut feelings to make decisions quickly and confidently. Start small (organic or standard baby wash?) and work up (should the TV be off while the baby's awake?). Quickly "try on" your decision before finalizing it. "See how you feel—relieved or rubbed the wrong way—and listen to yourself," says Debra Condren, Ph.D., a psychologist in New York. When you've made a choice, move on without second-guessing. "Keep reminding yourself: I'm top-dog expert here," Condren adds. (On the flip side, don't be rigid; if, down the road, you decide that a previous decision just doesn't work, so be it.)

6. TAKE NOTES. You may know the answers to all of the pediatrician's questions—from the number of bowel movements your baby has to her highest temperature—before you walk into his office, but once you're in there, you can barely remember your child's name. Research shows that people under acute stress have difficulty retaining information in their short-term memory. So bring notes to every appointment with your pediatrician and jot down the doctor's instructions while you're there. This might help you stay focused and view the doctor as a partner in your baby's health, rather than an intimidating authority figure.

7. DON'T HIDE YOUR EMOTIONS. As a new mom, it's understandable if you lose your calm after your baby has been on a crying jag for three hours or your toddler is throwing a tantrum in the supermarket. The surprise is, sometimes it's good for your baby to see you upset, as long as it's justified and doesn't happen too often.

As she grows, your child will look to you to learn how to handle emotions. When she sees you upset—whether it be sad, scared, mad or frustrated—tell her what's going on: "I

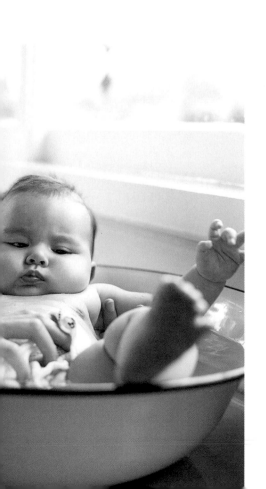

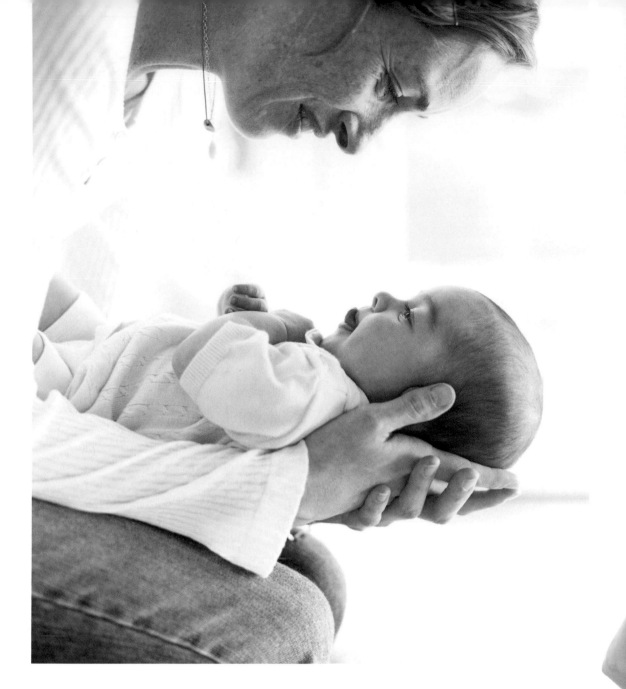

was feeling sad, but I feel better now" or "That was scary. I'm glad we're safe." Just dial back the drama if your baby starts to cry or look frightened.

8. BEWARE OF COMPETITIVE FRIENDS. Not even your mother-in-law can make you doubt yourself as much as that acquaintance whose child does everything first. Got a competitive friend who likes to dole out advice on how to get your baby to catch up, or who's fond of pointing out what you're doing wrong? Try this response: "We're happy with Sam's development, and so is his doctor."

9. TAKE TIME FOR YOU. "Taking a mom's day, hour or 15 minutes is required for good parenting," psychologist Yvonne Thomas says. "Parents need balance in their lives. If you don't have time to replenish your soul and rejuvenate yourself, you're not going to be at your best for your child. You're going to be impatient, frustrated and ill-tempered." Recharge your batteries by listening to soothing music or going out for a walk. You'll be a good role model for your child, showing her that taking care of yourself is a priority. (For more on how to be a good self-nurturer, see pg. 167.)

10. BE HAPPY TOGETHER. Spend as much undistracted time as you can with your baby, allowing yourself to be in the moment. Seeing your little one conquer a new milestone will remind you of the good job you're doing.

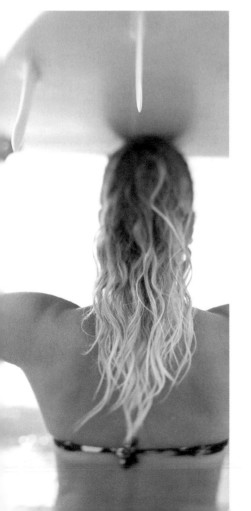

* As a new mom, it's important to take care of your needs, too. Go for a walk, listen to your favorite music or hit the surf— you'll be glad you did.

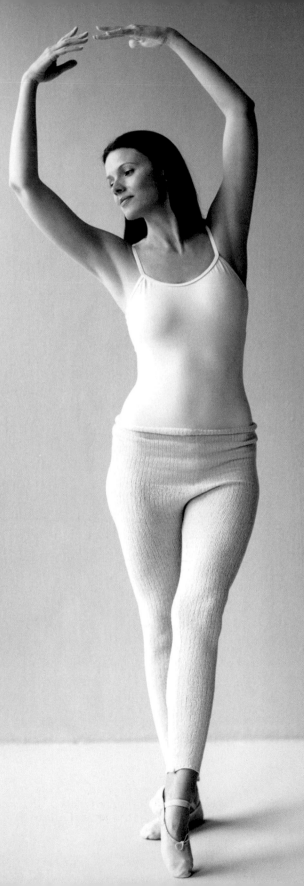

Prima mama
Build muscle—and your self-esteem—with this ballet-inspired workout.

Confidence stems from feeling—and looking—your best. As a new mom, you may be feeling slightly out of balance and less firm and fit than you did prepregnancy. A ballet-inspired workout is the perfect antidote, helping you regain stability and shed your excess baby weight while sculpting your legs, butt, arms, waistline and abdominal muscles. The following workout was designed by Jody Hoegstedt, creative director of Balletone, a ballet-based exercise program. "These graceful and effective moves will tone your entire body while improving posture and coordination," says Hoegstedt.

All you need to get started is a chair and workout band. Wait until six weeks after delivery before beginning this workout, slightly longer if you've had a Cesarean section. This routine can be done every other day, but always check with your doctor before beginning this or any exercise program.

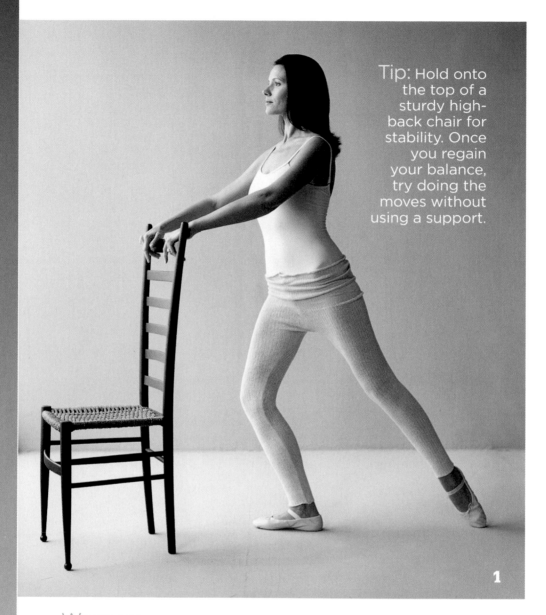

Tip: Hold onto the top of a sturdy high-back chair for stability. Once you regain your balance, try doing the moves without using a support.

1

Warm up **Warm up for 15 minutes by walking briskly, marching in place while doing opposite knee-to-elbow knee lifts, or dancing around the room to your favorite music.**

1 CIRCLES BACK Face the back of a chair and hold it with both hands at arm's distance, feet turned out and abs pulled in. Point and slide your left toe forward, then circle it to the left and back as you bend your right knee and lean your torso slightly forward [shown]. Straighten your right leg as you sweep your left toe in a circle back to starting position. Complete 5 to 10 circles, then switch legs.

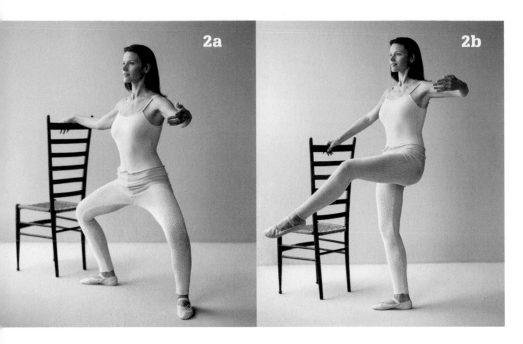

2a

2b

2

PLIÉ WITH ATTITUDE
Stand holding the chair back with your right hand, legs wider than hip distance, feet turned out and abs tight. Bend your knees while lowering your hips into a plié. Squeeze your glutes (butt) to help steady your pelvis [A]. Straighten your legs and lift your left leg to hip height. Your lifted knee should be turned out in an "attitude" position [B]. Return to plié. Complete 5 to 10 reps, then switch sides and repeat.

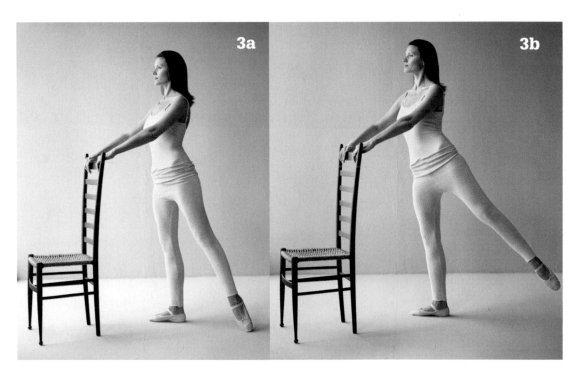

3a

3b

3   **MOVING ARABESQUE** Face the back of a chair and hold it with both hands at arm's distance, feet hip-width apart and slightly turned out, abs tight. Shift your weight to your right foot and point your left toe back, maintaining straight legs [A]. Keeping your hips still, lift your left leg a few inches off the floor into an arabesque. Squeeze your glutes and keep your shoulders back and down [B]. Slowly lower your left toe to the floor, ending in starting position. Complete 5 to 10 lifts, then switch legs.

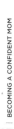

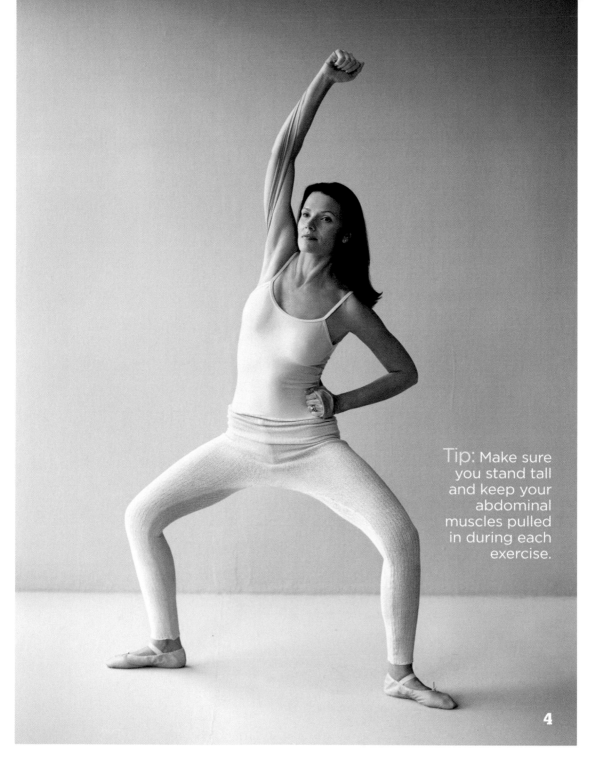

Tip: Make sure you stand tall and keep your abdominal muscles pulled in during each exercise.

4

4 SIDE STRETCH WITH OVERHEAD RAISE Stand with your feet wider than hip distance, feet and knees turned out comfortably from the hips, abs tight. Place a workout band across your lower back, holding an end in each hand and wrapped around your palm, elbows bent and hands on hips. Bend your knees into a plié as you lean your torso to the left and raise your right arm overhead [shown]. Straighten your legs and lower your right hand to starting position. Complete 5 to 10 reps, then switch sides.

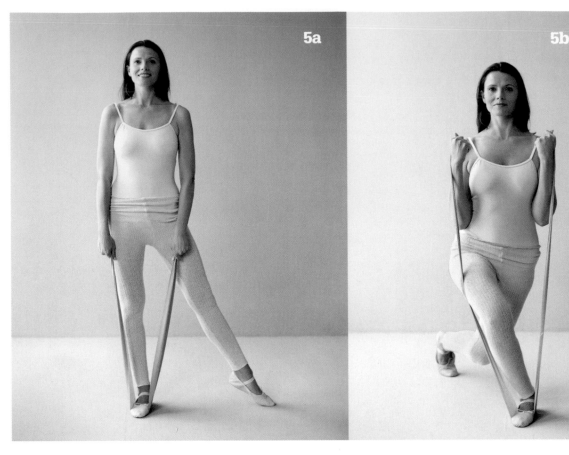

5a   5b

5 **CURTSY LUNGE WITH BICEP CURL** Stand with the middle of the band under your right foot and point your left foot to the side. Hold one end of the band in each hand, arms at your sides, palms facing your thighs [A]. Step your left foot behind your right at an angle and bend your knees in a curtsy as you bend your elbows and curl your arms toward your chest [B]. Slowly straighten your arms and legs and return to starting position. Complete 5 to 10 reps, then switch sides.

* This dance-inspired workout will help you regain stability and shed your excess baby weight while sculpting your legs, arms, waistline and abs.

6 BALLET SIT-UPS WITH CURL Sit on the floor with your knees bent and feet together. Wrap the band around your feet, then bring the ends between your knees. Lie back with your knees open, sides of feet touching the floor, arms straight and fingers reaching toward your knees. Bend your elbows as you curl your head and shoulders off the floor into a crunch, bringing your fists toward your chest in a bicep curl [shown]. Slowly straighten your arms as you curl your torso down to the floor. Complete 5 to 10 reps.

Cool down Cool down for five minutes by stretching your lower back, legs and hips, holding each stretch for at least 30 seconds without bouncing.

Tip: Keep strong tension on the band throughout the entire exercise.

6

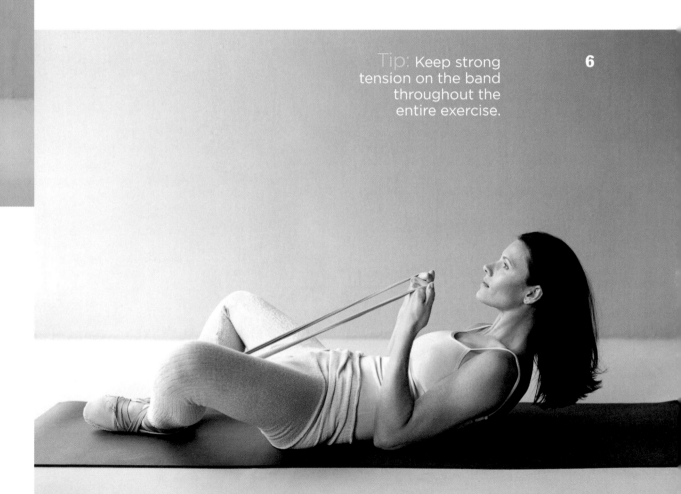

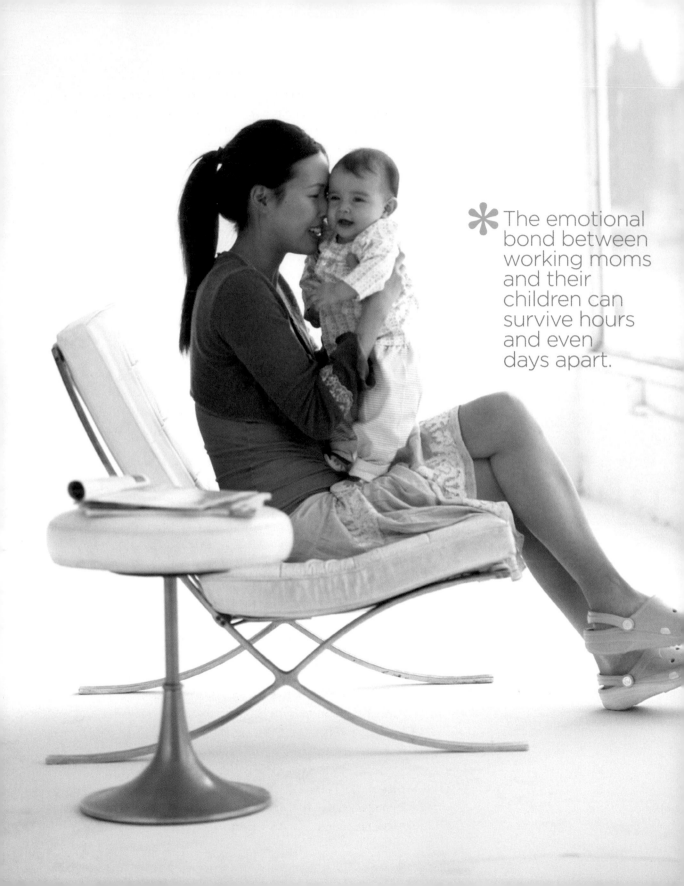

*The emotional bond between working moms and their children can survive hours and even days apart.

Return policy

Consider a gradual return to your job to make the transition easier for you and your baby. One fact that will boost your negotiating power with your boss is that it costs between 75 percent and 200 percent of your salary to replace you—strong incentive for your employer to accommodate your requests. A few options:

START OFF PART TIME
Work three or four days a week for the first month back.

BE FLEXIBLE
Arrange your schedule to allow you more time with your baby during waking hours—for example, work from 7 a.m. to 3 p.m.

EAT AT YOUR DESK
Work through lunch so that you can head home an hour earlier at the end of the day.

FIND A WORK BUDDY
Share a job with a co-worker, each of you working part time.

Going back to work after baby

If you are contemplating a return to your job after weeks or months of maternity leave, be forewarned: You may be bombarded with intense and unexpected emotions, ranging from profound sadness to guilt to deep relief. The spectrum of reactions is common—and normal. "Some women who have spent their entire adult lives building a career they love suddenly have no desire to return to work," says Susan Walker-Matthews, Ph.D., a clinical psychologist specializing in women's health services and pediatric psychology at Charleston Area Medical Center's Women and Children's Hospital in Charleston, W. Va. Yet the reverse is also true. "Other women worry because they return to work easily and don't know what they would do with their children—or themselves—if they were at home all day," Walker-Matthews adds.

The reality of having a new baby can change your goals and perspective dramatically. Whether your idea was to return to work or to stay home, the "perfect" plan you had while pregnant may seem all wrong once you're holding your baby—and you're now a new mom.

GIVE YOURSELF A BREAK Working mothers may be blindsided by their emotions at the end of maternity leave because they've been so consumed by the practical matters of lining up day care, figuring out schedules and planning for emergencies. And even if they do see the emotional tidal wave coming, where do they run for cover? Support can be hard to find in a society that tends to frown on the full-time working mother, even if she has no choice.

"When a woman faces the issue of going back to work, she triggers layers of social, personal and familial expectations that may be unrealistic for her and her family," says Walker-Matthews. "This can be difficult." While suffering separation from their babies, many working moms also berate themselves with the outdated notion that the only good mother is the one who stays home full time with her child. Yet a child will sense his mother's love and internalize her presence, experts say. That's why the emotional bond between working moms and their children can survive hours and even days apart.

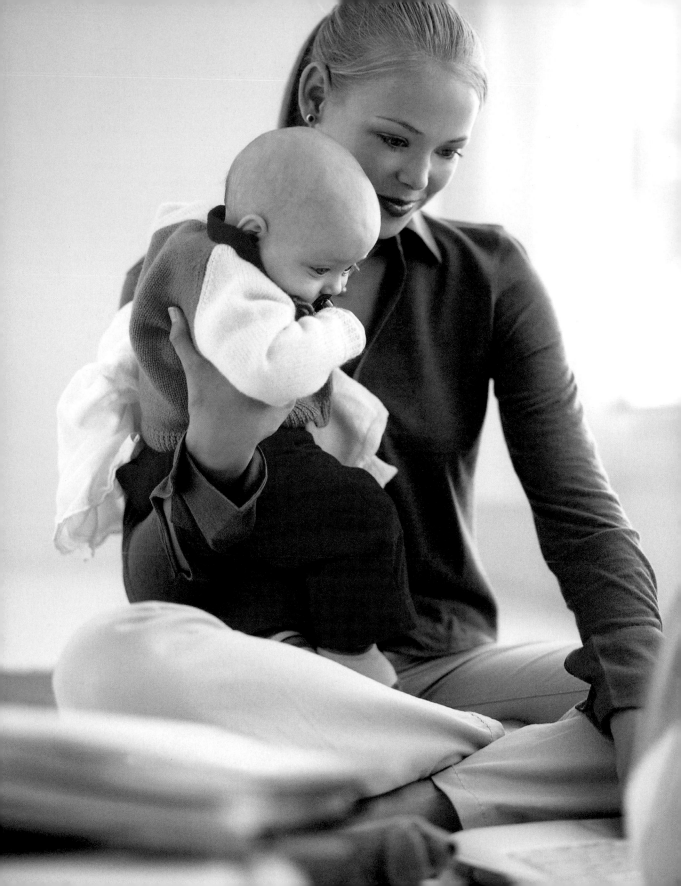

CONSIDER YOUR OPTIONS Alternatives for women who want to spend more time with their children include working from home a few days a week, negotiating a leave from the job, choosing a day-care center near their workplace so that they can visit during the day, working part time, or switching to a career that allows more flexibility or provides on-site day care. Some companies even let parents bring their children to work on slower days.

While every woman's experience is different, the emotion that unifies nearly all new moms is guilt. One way to ease the guilt is to create a work schedule you feel is best for you and your baby—and be willing to make adjustments along the way (for tips, see "Return Policy," pg. 163). Also keep photos of your baby with you at the office and, if possible, call your caregiver a few times during the day just to check in—doing so will help you feel more connected to your child. And consider a later bedtime for your baby so that you can spend more family time together.

Whether you burst into tears when you get to work or breathe a sigh of relief, go easy on yourself. Unlike other jobs, there are no "right" choices in motherhood. As Walker-Matthews says: "Have a sense of reality, and don't get too dogmatic about trying to do everything perfectly."

Working moms manage better

You'd think the effort of mothering a baby would subtract from your productiveness at work, but being a caring and involved parent could make you a more effective employee. In a study of male and female managers, those who were most committed to family life and raising their children were also rated highest in job performance by their peers, bosses and subordinates.

"As a parent, you learn to multitask, manage your emotions and resolve conflict," says study co-author Laura Graves, Ph.D., an associate professor of management at Clark University in Worcester, Mass. "Those skills are also valuable at work." Another bonus moms and dads bring to the office is a greater satisfaction with life—good feelings that enhance your mood on the job. "The popular press and television often focus on the stressors that children bring, but for most of us, the positives of helping your kids develop outweigh the negatives," Graves says.

However, there's no denying that it's tricky trying to juggle workplace obligations and baby care. To lighten your load, Graves suggests you prioritize what's most important, and moderate your expectations accordingly. Finally, relax. Your childless colleagues probably think you're doing a great job.

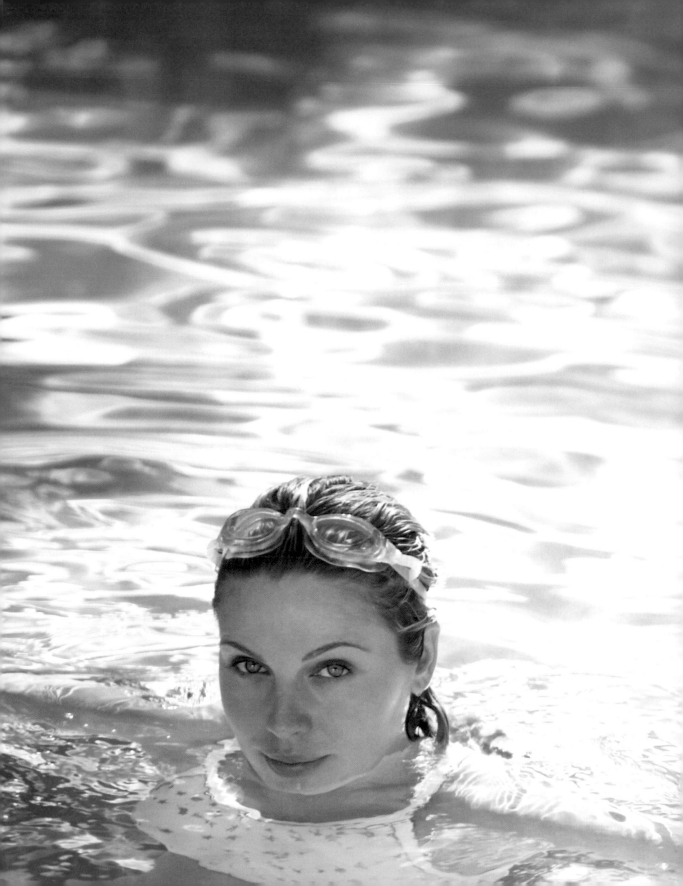

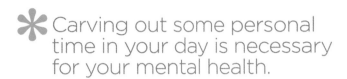
Carving out some personal time in your day is necessary for your mental health.

Make space for me-time

At some point during your pregnancy, you may have thought: How can I give up chatty lunches with friends, leisurely candlelit dinners and spontaneous shopping trips? But that was then. Now you know exactly how fast a new mother can downsize her wish list from a romantic weekend getaway to a few minutes of free time to take a shower, sip a cup of tea or read a magazine.

Some aspects of your life have indeed changed forever. But the sooner you can recapture a few pre-baby routines, the sooner you and your infant will reap the benefits. "You're a better mother to your kids if you take care of yourself," says Karen Kleiman, M.S.W., executive director of The Postpartum Stress Center in Rosemont, Pa. She advises new moms to integrate favorite activities back into their schedules as soon as the timing feels realistic. You need to do things that make you happy, even if they're as simple as pruning the rosebushes or going to your book club. Yes, you'll face logistical obstacles, but as veteran moms will attest, a little planning goes a long way.

BANISH THE GUILT Before you can even think about organizing some time apart from your baby, you need to stop seeing it as self-indulgence. "Our society holds impossible standards for the 'ideal' mother," Kleiman says. "She's selfless, endlessly patient and devoted to putting her children first to the exclusion of everything else in her life."

If you've internalized this image of perfection, taking an hour out for a jog or a manicure can feel selfish. But no one can keep on giving without replenishing the inner well. If you don't participate in activities that make you feel whole, you won't be happy and relaxed enough to fully engage with your child. Too much deprivation, notes Kleiman, can lead to feelings of resentment, even meltdowns (yours, followed closely by your baby's).

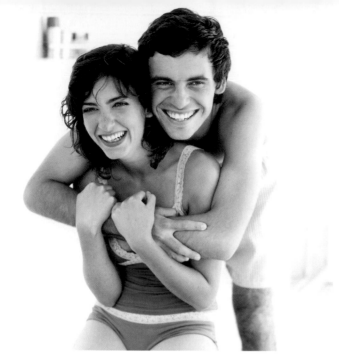

COUPLE UP Whether you go out together once a week or once a month, spending time alone with your partner reinforces your family's strong foundation. Schedule a date with your partner—and hire a babysitter.

DON'T WAIT If exercise—or reading or gardening—was a priority before your baby arrived, find time for it now, too. It's crucial to rekindle your passions early on, rather than waiting until your infant reaches developmental milestones—such as sleeping through the night or weaning—that you imagine will make your life more manageable.

THINK OUTSIDE THE BOX In a haze of sleep deprivation, the obstacles to finding time for yourself can seem more insurmountable than they really are. Look for creative solutions. Can't go to the gym for lack of a regular babysitter? Find a gym that offers infant care, as many YMCAs do, or invest in a stair-stepper or a good stroller for walking. Need occasional free time to maintain friendships or to keep up with work contacts? Initiate a baby swap with a friend.

Even with prioritizing, getting your life back takes time. Acknowledging this is half the battle. As Kleiman tells new parents, "The postpartum period requires three attributes: patience, realistic expectations and resilience." Sounds like the essential ingredients for high-quality parenting.

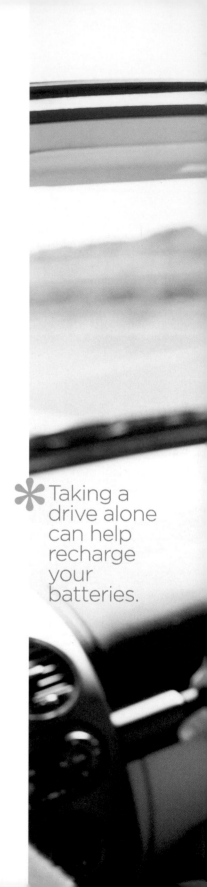

*Taking a drive alone can help recharge your batteries.

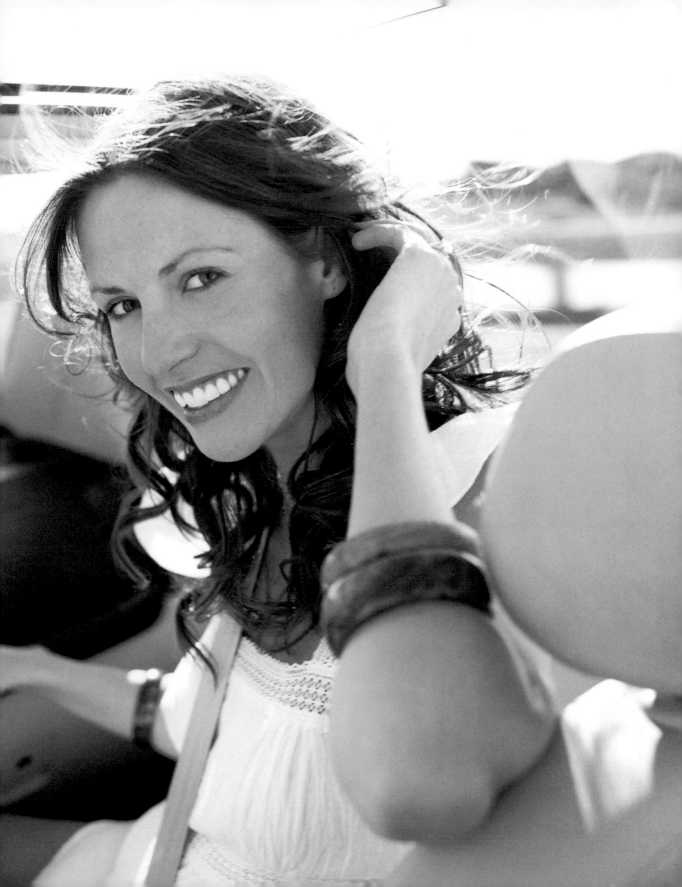

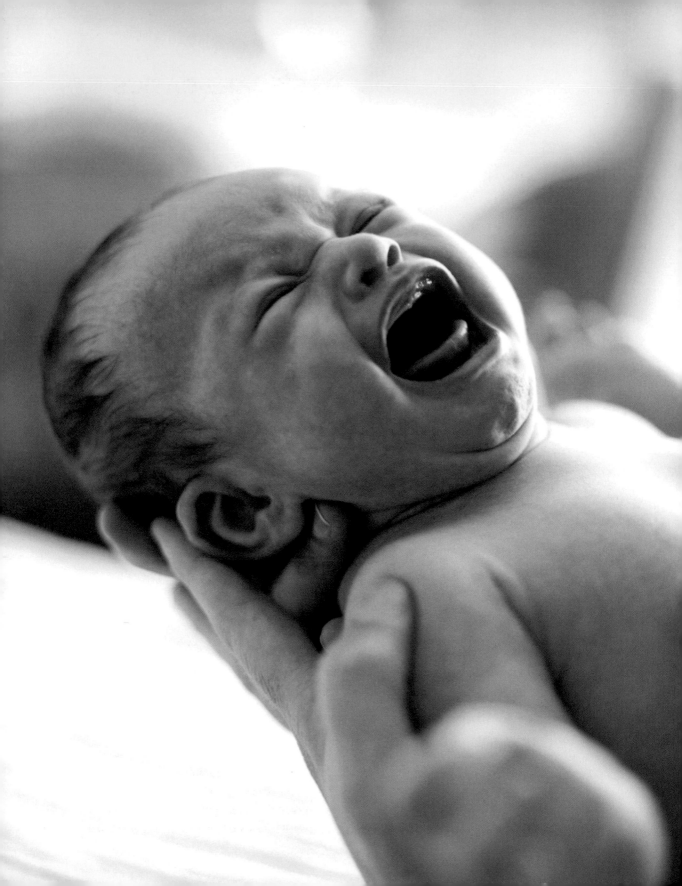

Taking care of a newborn can be challenging.

Many new parents worry that they won't know what to do when it comes time to give their baby her first bath or soothe a crying infant. The good news? The most basic baby-care tasks are just that: basic. Once you get the hang of washing a slippery baby or tending to a sick infant, you'll soon be able to do it without thinking twice.

  From that first diaper change to first fever, the following guide to caring for your infant will make you a baby-care pro in no time. Plus, learning the best ways to care for your baby's body—from head to tiny toes—will help keep him happy, healthy and well.

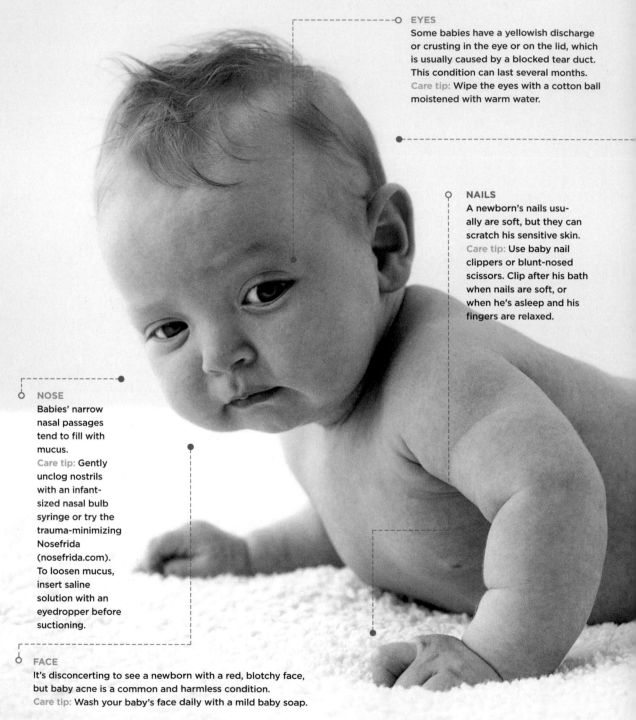

Your newborn: a user's guide

Here are some pediatrician-approved tips for keeping your baby clean and healthy from head to toe.

EYES

Some babies have a yellowish discharge or crusting in the eye or on the lid, which is usually caused by a blocked tear duct. This condition can last several months. **Care tip:** Wipe the eyes with a cotton ball moistened with warm water.

NAILS

A newborn's nails usually are soft, but they can scratch his sensitive skin. **Care tip:** Use baby nail clippers or blunt-nosed scissors. Clip after his bath when nails are soft, or when he's asleep and his fingers are relaxed.

NOSE

Babies' narrow nasal passages tend to fill with mucus. **Care tip:** Gently unclog nostrils with an infant-sized nasal bulb syringe or try the trauma-minimizing Nosefrida (nosefrida.com). To loosen mucus, insert saline solution with an eyedropper before suctioning.

FACE

It's disconcerting to see a newborn with a red, blotchy face, but baby acne is a common and harmless condition. **Care tip:** Wash your baby's face daily with a mild baby soap.

HEAD

Many newborns develop a scaly scalp condition called cradle cap. It typically disappears in the first few months.

Care tip: Wash your baby's hair with a gentle baby shampoo no more than three times a week and gently brush out the scales daily using a baby hairbrush or soft toothbrush.

BOTTOM

Too much moisture plus sensitive skin can equal diaper rash for many babies.

Care tip: Change diapers frequently. Rinse your baby's bottom with water during each change and blot dry. Avoid using wipes; they may irritate skin. Barrier creams, such as petroleum jelly or white zinc oxide, may help.

LEGS

Newborns' legs are bowed out and the feet are turned in, which is no surprise, given their previous cramped living quarters.

Care tip: Don't worry about it—your baby's legs and feet will straighten in anywhere from six to 18 months.

SKIN

Some babies develop red, itchy patches called eczema or atopic dermatitis— an inheritable skin condition. Care tip: Limit baths to 10 minutes, and use a mild, fragrance-free soap and lukewarm water; liberally apply hypoallergenic skin cream immediately afterward. Stick to cotton clothing.

UMBILICAL CORD

Keep the umbilical cord stump clean and dry; it will shrivel and fall off within a few weeks.

Care tip: Avoid covering the cord area with a diaper and stick to sponge baths until the stump detaches.

CIRCUMCISION

The tip of his penis will be swollen, and a yellow scab will appear.

Care tip: Gently clean the genital area with warm water daily. Use petroleum jelly to protect the site and prevent his penis from sticking to a diaper.

Mastering the essentials

There's a first time for everything and caring for a newborn is no exception. Here, time-tested and mother-approved tips to making each baby-care "first" a success:

The first diaper change

WHAT YOU'LL NEED: clean diaper, diaper ointment, cotton balls or washcloth, warm water. (Since many baby wipes contain cleansing agents that are irritating to your baby's bottom, experts recommend that you wait a month before using them on delicate newborn skin.)

HOW TO CHANGE A DIAPER

LAY THE BABY ON HIS BACK on the changing table; keep a firm hand on him at all times so that he can't roll off.

REMOVE THE DIRTY DIAPER and roll it up. If you have a boy, keep a cloth diaper or washcloth handy to place over his penis so that he doesn't pee on himself—or you!

WIPE FROM FRONT TO BACK with cotton balls or a washcloth and lukewarm water. (Plush paper towels work, too.)

LET HIM AIR-DRY FOR A MOMENT, then apply diaper ointment if he has a rash. Tuck the back of the clean diaper under his bottom, pull the front between his legs and fasten.

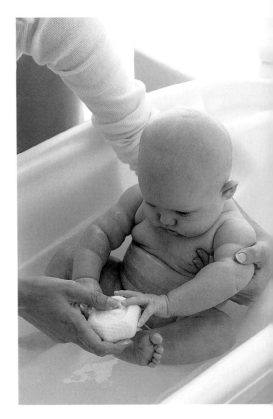

The first real bath

WHAT YOU'LL NEED: baby bathtub (a clean sink will do), washcloth, baby soap and shampoo, plastic cup, hooded towel. (Stick to sponge baths until the umbilical cord stump falls off, usually within the first few weeks.)

HOW TO GIVE YOUR BABY A BATH

MAKE SURE the room is warm and cozy.

FILL THE BABY'S TUB with a few inches of warm water. Test the water temperature using your elbow or the inside of your wrist, and have your supplies within reach.

EASE HIM INTO THE TUB gradually, feet first; he may startle, so lean him backward gently, keeping your arm around his back. Hold him securely under his armpit.

WASH HIS BODY FIRST, paying attention to the genital area, behind the ears, and the folds under the arms and neck.

WASH HIS HAIR LAST so that he doesn't get cold.

USE A CUP TO RINSE his entire body with warm water.

WRAP HIM in a warm hooded towel to dry off.

*As long as you're doing a good job of cleaning your baby's diaper area, two or three baths a week are all he needs.

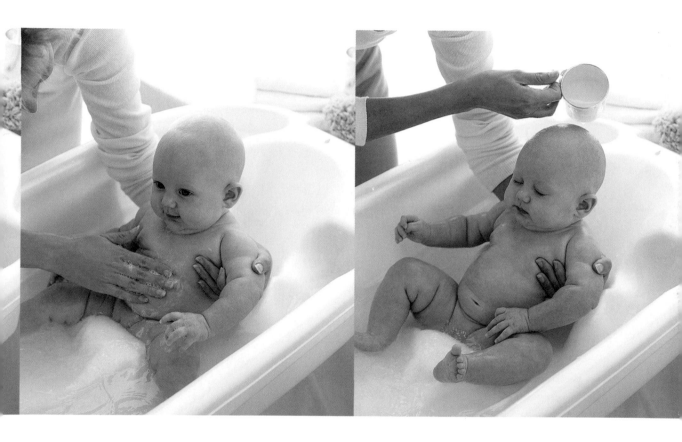

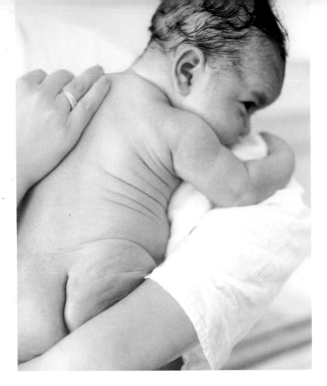

The first fever

WHAT YOU'LL NEED: digital rectal thermometer (the most accurate type for infants), petroleum jelly.

HOW TO TAKE YOUR BABY'S TEMPERATURE

DIP THE END of the thermometer into the petroleum jelly.

LAY THE BABY ON HIS BELLY, and slowly insert the thermometer just past the tip into his rectum.

GENTLY PRESS his buttock checks closed for one to two minutes, then remove the thermometer.

The first crying jag

WHAT YOU'LL NEED: loving arms, patience, a soothing voice.

HOW TO COMFORT A CRYING BABY

RULE OUT THE OBVIOUS potential causes: Check to see if the baby's diaper is soiled, if he's too hot or cold, or if his diaper or clothing is pinching his skin.

LET HIM SUCK ON YOUR BREAST, a bottle, your finger or a pacifier. (Babies have an intense need to suck.)

RE-CREATE A WOMBLIKE ENVIRONMENT by swaddling him securely in a blanket with his arms tucked inside. Then hold him snugly on his left side or stomach and jiggle him gently while making "shushing" sounds.

GET MOVING Walk, rock, jiggle, sway, take a car ride or put him in an infant swing. (Babies love motion!)